Thueson's Guide to
OVER-THE-COUNTER
DRUGS

A Symptom-by-Symptom Handbook of the Best Nonprescription Drugs

DAVID O. THUESON, Ph.D.

NEW HARBINGER PUBLICATIONS, INC

Publishers Note

This publication is designed to provide accurate and authoritative information in regard to the subject matter covered. It is sold with the understanding that the publisher is not engaged in rendering psychological, financial, legal, or other professional services. If expert assistance or counseling is needed, the services of a competent professional should be sought.

Cover design by SHELBY DESIGNS & ILLUSTRATES.
Text design by Tracy Marie Powell.

ISBN 1-57224-006-7

Originally published as *The Best "OTC" Drugs for Self-Care* by Abat Pathos Publishing, La Jolla, California.

Printed in the United States of America

Writing this book has been a labor of love. It is intended to help many, but was made possible by the patience, support, and encouragement of a few and is dedicated to them, my family.

Quick Reference Chart

Symptoms	page	Acetominophen	Aspirin	Benzocaine	Benzoyl Peroxide	Caffeine	Carboxymethylcellulose	Chlorpheniramine	Clotrimazole	Dextromethorphan	Dibucaine	Diphenhydramine	Dyclonine
		19	20	38	113	21	166	69	139	54	38	55	38
Acne	112				114								
Allergy	68		75					70				69	
Arthritis	29												
Athlete's foot	138								140				
Backache	30	30	30										
Bacterial infections	119												
Burns/bites/stings	124			44									
Colds	50	66											
Congestion	61	66						73					
Constipation	95												
Cough	54									64			
Dandruff	129												
Diarrhea	89												
Dry eye	166						167						
Dry skin	136												
Flu	65	66								66			
Hangover	106												
Headache	32	22								65			
Heartburn, indigestion, ulcers	81												
Hemorrhoids	92			93							93		
Menstrual symptoms	180					184							
Nasal/sinus congestion	56												
Nausea	86												
Pain & fever	17	22	27							65			
Poison ivy/oak/sumac	144												
Red, irritated eyes	169												
Sinus headache	56	66											
Skin rash/allergy	115							160					
Sleep aids	174	172										175	
Sore throat	52												40
Sprains	35												
Sunburn	153			44									
Vaginal itching	188			190					191				
Wounds & injuries	156												

Guiafenisen	Hydrocortisone	Ibuprofen	Loperamide	Mag/Al Hydroxide	Meclizine	Methylcellulose	Miconazole	Naphazoline	Naproxen Sodium	Oxymetazoline	Pamabrom	Petrolatum	Phenolphthalein	Polymyxin	Pseudoephedrine	Selenium Sulfide	Zinc Oxide
55	39	20	90	82	86	96	139	167	20	61	181	93	97	120	57	130	93
		73													72		
							140										
		30															
														121			
		65													65		
64		65													64		
				102		99						100					
64		65													64		
																131	
			91														
											137						
		106															
		65													65		
				83													
												93					93
		182									184						
										62					58		
					87												
		21													65		
	146																
								170		170							
		59													59		
117																	124
		176															
		35															
	153	161															
	188						191										
														157			

Table of Contents

About the Author

Dr. David O. Thueson, Ph.D., is a medical scientist, inventor, author, and educator. He earned his Bachelor of Science degree in 1971 with a premedicine major, and in 1976 was awarded a Ph.D. in Pharmacology from the University of Utah. After two years of post-doctoral training in the Department of Internal Medicine, Dave joined the faculty of the University of Texas Medical Branch. He taught medical and graduate students and physicians. He conducted research, focusing on allergic diseases and asthma, for another five years. In 1982, Dave joined the Parke-Davis Pharmaceutical Company where he directed the asthma, allergy, and respiratory drug discovery programs. After six years with Parke-Davis, he became Director of Pharmacology for a small biotech pharmaceutical company, specializing in designing new drugs for immune-inflammatory diseases (such as asthma, arthritis, allergies). He has authored more than 45 articles in medical journals and books and holds several U.S. and foreign patents. Dave's interests, expertise, and desire to improve self-care led him to write this book and to promote consumer education. His goals are to increase public awareness of over-the-counter drugs, their proper use, effectiveness, and safety.

Note to Readers

This book is designed to provide scientifically sound information with regard to the subject matter covered. It is sold with the understanding that the publisher and author are not engaged in rendering professional medical advice for the diagnosis or treatment of disease or illness. If expert medical advice is required, the services of a competent medical professional should be sought.

It is not the purpose of this book to provide all of the information that is available to the author or publisher, but to summarize, clarify, amplify, and supplement other sources of information available to the public. You are urged to read additional material and learn as much as you can about self-care of minor symptoms, illnesses, and disease to more clearly understand the need for, and how to use, nonprescription drugs.

Self-care is not the answer to all health problems, illnesses, or disease, and good judgment must be exercised in order to determine when to self-treat and when to seek treatment from a physician or other licensed health-care professional. Only you can make this determination on the basis of your experience and understanding, and you must accept the risks associated with whatever choice you make.

Every effort has been made to make this book as complete and accurate as possible. However, **there may be mistakes**, both typographical and in content. Therefore, this book should only be used as a general guide and not as the ultimate source of health-care information for self-treatment. Furthermore, this manual only contains information available up to the publishing date, and newer or more accurate information may now be available.

Each individual product contains more detailed and up-to-date information and instructions, **which should always be fol-**

lowed. The author and New Harbinger Publications shall have neither liability nor responsibility to any person or entity with respect
to any loss or damage caused, or alleged to be caused, directly or
indirectly, by the information contained in this book.

1

Introduction

Over-the-counter drugs are medicines that you can buy without a doctor's prescription. Our modern (U.S. government-approved and regulated) over-the-counter drugs are quite safe and effective medicines for the self-treatment of minor illnesses and various symptoms. They are available in drug stores, in most supermarkets, and many other retail outlets. Not only are over-the-counter drugs useful for the treatment of unpleasant symptoms, but in some cases even curative agents are available for self-care without a prescription. Many of these medicines are former prescription-only drugs that have been changed to over-the-counter availability during the past several years by the USFDA (U. S. Food and Drug Administration). Many more drugs that are currently prescription-only are now under review, or are being considered by sponsoring companies for over-the-counter use within the next few years. This has occurred as a direct result of demands by the U.S. population for a greater role in health maintenance and reduced costs for medical care. The ever increasing level of consumer sophistication and knowledge makes self-care ever more practical and effective, thereby increasing the need for access to safe and effective medicines without a doctor's intervention, in order to maintain and improve our quality of life.

Modern over-the-counter medicines:

- Are safe and effective drugs that can be used to treat a variety of illnesses and symptoms.

- Save you time and money by reducing visits to the doctor when you have minor symptoms or illnesses.

- Are less toxic (safer) than prescription medicines and frequently are just as effective.

- Can reduce the length of your illness and the discomfort and suffering involved.

- Provide immediate relief of symptoms while you are trying to get in to see your doctor.

Most people do not want to limit their activities because of minor symptoms, and only do so when discomfort is great. We are too busy to spend a day in bed except when we are really ill. The appropriate use of over-the-counter drugs can reduce symptoms; nearly always without any deleterious effect on the illness or on the speed of recovery.

Over-the-counter drugs are critical elements in our health-care system, both in terms of the economic benefits (savings) and the health maintenance aspects for our society. Some have been used for many years, while others are recent additions to self-care because the USFDA switched them from prescription-only to over-the-counter status. Just this year, *naproxen sodium* (a pain reliever and antiarthritis drug with the brand name Aleve) was switched. A few years ago *ibuprofen* (similar to aspirin) and *clotrimazole* (for yeast infections) were also changed to over-the-counter from prescription-only availability. Many other examples could be listed. If many over-the-counter drugs were still only available by prescription, health-care costs would be even more astronomical than they are. Most estimates are that 70% to 90% of all illnesses are self-treated. We spend billions of dollars every year to treat ourselves, to maintain our well-being, to relieve common symptoms, and cure minor illnesses. Self-care dramatically reduces the burden on the health-care system. Without this benefit, the costs and increased patient load would escalate tremendously. If only 2% of people using over-the-counter drugs visited their doctors instead of treating themselves, the wasted time, additional medical facilities required, number of additional physicians needed, and wasted use of sophisticated training on minor ailments would amount to hundreds of millions of dollars each year.

Proper use of over-the-counter drugs saves money and reduces stress on the already overburdened health-care system. In addition, it reduces the dollar cost of care and saves additional health problems that result from the excessive and inappropriate use of prescription drugs. Many doctors prescribe these powerful, toxic drugs unnecessarily, costing more money, and causing more adverse drug reactions. In contrast, over-the-counter drug purchases amount to less than two cents of every health-care dollar spent in the United States; but the benefit is immeasurable, especially when you consider the impact on reducing the time lost from school and work, fewer doctor visits, less prescription drug use, lower insurance costs, and tax savings for the care of the poor and elderly.

Why This Book?

There are hundreds of thousands of over-the-counter medicines on store shelves. How can someone choose from so many options? Especially when there is also a shortage of understandable, accurate information upon which to base a judgment. The purpose of this book is to give the average person the information needed to objectively evaluate, choose, and use properly the best drug for the self-treatment of common symptoms and minor diseases. This information will permit you to manage many illnesses and avoid the time, cost, and inconvenience of a visit to your doctor (or urgent care or emergency room). This information will also be valuable for the temporary treatment of minor symptoms until you can be seen by a doctor.

With this book you will:

- Never again have to guess which medicine to use or rely on misleading advertising claims to choose.

- Learn which over-the-counter medicines are safe and effective and how to use them to their fullest advantage.

- Save money on doctor visits and medicines.

- Have options for treatment if you have special needs or problems or can't use the first choice.

- Know more than the professionals you would usually consult for help (doctor, pharmacist, or nurse) about over-the-counter medicines and their use.

Thousands of pieces of information and hundreds of comparative studies have been consulted, reviewed, and evaluated to determine which drug or drugs in each class are the safest and most effective. Many problems that can be effectively self-treated go untreated because of the lack of information about a product that works. In many cases consumers have previously tried over-the-counter drugs which were not effective, and have given up the search for effective over-the-counter medications. This book details alternatives and options and recommends first choice agents that benefit the majority of people. Second, and sometimes third, choices are given in case you happen to be one of the minority who isn't helped or has undesirable side effects when the first choice agent is used.

If you are one of today's typical well-informed and educated consumers, you are more interested in your own health than ever before. As individuals and as a society, we want and demand more involvement and information about our health and feel more responsible for our own care. Our education allows us more freedom and the opportunity to take charge and make a difference in controlling our quality of life. With this book as a guide, you can confidently evaluate, select, and use over-the-counter medicines to make a genuine difference in your health and well-being and prevent and treat the illnesses we all occasionally encounter.

Do Over-the-Counter Drugs Really Work?

Yes, there is no question that most over-the-counter drugs are effective for their intended purpose. In fact, any drugs that are not both effective and safe will soon be off the market completely. Initially, hundreds of drugs (active ingredients) were "grandfathered" into use at the time the U.S. government first began regulating drugs. Some drugs were made available only on the order of a physician, and others were allowed to be sold to the public. The real difference between over-the-counter and prescription drugs is not related to their effectiveness or potency differences, but to the safety of their use. Most prescription drugs are controlled by doctors because of the frequency and/or severity of toxic side effects associated with their use. A few require special knowledge or training or special tests to diagnose the disease for their use, and therefore would not be useful for self-care anyway.

Until 30 years ago most people, including medical professionals, believed that over-the-counter drugs were ineffective. Some were also thought to be unsafe, poor substitutes for prescription medicines. This concept was partially accurate, but is a holdover from the days of "patent medicines." Nearly all patent medicines were either alcohol disguised as medicine, or elixirs of addicting opiates, such as codeine and morphine. These were subsequently tightly regulated by the USFDA for use only under the direction and supervision of a doctor, and have not been legally available for many years, except by prescription.

Some 20 years ago the USFDA began a detailed and comprehensive review of all over-the-counter drugs. Only those ingredients proven in human use to be both safe and effective will be allowed to remain on the market when the reviews are complete. Many hundreds of unsafe or ineffective drugs have already been declared illegal and removed from sale. As it currently stands, the list of safe and effective ingredients permitted in over-the-counter products numbers a few hundred, down from the more than 1,000 ingredients formerly available and claimed to be effective and safe. However, even though hundreds of ineffective or unsafe ingredients have already been removed and more will soon no longer be available, the estimated number of products (primarily different brands) containing just the approved ingredients, or combinations of approved ingredients, is currently estimated at more than 300,000.

In many cases there are several drugs in each category of drug activity that are both safe and effective. The typical consumer is understandably often unable to make informed decisions about which agent is the best and which one to use for a particular indication.

The main purpose of this self-help guide is to provide information in order to promote the proper use of over-the-counter
drugs in maintaining the quality of life and health when self-treatment is desired and is appropriate and safe. The over-the-counter
drugs recommended in this book have been thoroughly tested and
proven effective in comparative studies with other drugs or against
a placebo (a lookalike but inactive twin of the drug), usually in
tests where the observers (health professionals) were not aware of
what the patient took. In this testing, using a "blinded" design,
neither the patients nor observers know which patients are given
the placebo and which are given the authentic drug. After the treatment results are determined, the effectiveness of the drug and placebo are compared.

Are Over-the-Counter Drugs Safe?

No drug is completely safe since they are all intended to modify
body functions, correct problems, or cure illnesses. There is a potential to do harm as well as good. The risk is present, but low,
especially when over-the-counter medicines are taken as directed.
Over-the-counter drugs are available primarily because they have
been shown to be quite safe, after years of experience and widespread use. When used as directed, the benefits clearly exceed the
risk. Even if side effects occur when these medicines are used, they
are rarely serious and almost always quickly disappear when use
of the drug is discontinued.

Do Over-the-Counter Drugs
Save Money?

Yes, especially compared to prescription drugs, over-the-counter
drugs are a real bargain. The savings to the health-care system are
so great they are impossible to estimate accurately. In many cases
these drugs also save the time and money spent on a visit to the
doctor's office. Reduced side effects are also an important consideration in their advantages.

Over-the-counter drugs also contribute to our overall quality of life by reducing pain and suffering and helping us to be

productive at times when we might otherwise be unable to do anything but rest and suffer with unpleasant symptoms.

Additional significant cost savings can be realized when using over-the-counter drugs by knowing that advertised brands are much more expensive than the generic equivalent, but that the ingredients (and effectiveness) are nearly always the same. Often, more than half the cost of brand name over-the-counter drugs results from advertising expenses that are added to the drug's cost. Although slight differences may occur, the government regulates the purity, strength, and dosage of over-the-counter drugs so that generic and brand names are essentially identical.

An Additional Benefit of Over-the-Counter Drugs

Besides contributing to our overall well-being and reducing medical costs significantly, over-the-counter drugs have other benefits that may not be as obvious. One of the most important is the amount of information printed on the label. Over-the-counter drugs have complete written instructions for use; information on appropriate indications; and cautions about side effects, drug interactions, and how long they should be used. Usually, prescription drugs have very little information; and verbal instructions are often given, which are frequently unclear, incomplete, or very complicated and quickly forgotten.

How Do You Choose Among Over-the-Counter Drugs?

Of course there are many options and possibilities when it comes to choosing the "right drug" for your situation. Surveys have found that many people rely on a doctor, pharmacist, or nurse for advice. Others consult family members or friends, are persuaded by advertising, by reading labels, or they just try things until they find something that works.

Unfortunately, none of these sources is optimal. Most health professionals are not very knowledgeable about the range of over-the-counter products or how to choose among them. It is exceedingly rare to find even a well-trained professional who has read any of the scientific medical literature comparing different over-the-counter ingredients, or who has the information to objectively judge the relative benefits and costs of the ingredients, let alone know which brands contain them.

Another problem is conflict of interest. In recommending over-the-counter agents, many health professionals feel they deprive themselves of their own livelihood by reducing patient visits, prescriptions, and other care-giving activities that generate their income. It is also widely recognized that the medical profession as a whole organizes itself to oppose proposed drug switches from prescription-only to over the counter, ostensibly on the grounds of scientific and humanitarian (safety) issues, when the fear of loss of fees is in fact the major motivation. Many more over-the-counter agents could be available if not for this opposition.

This book arms you with the information you need to make wise choices among over-the-counter drugs. You will learn to recognize their basic (generic) ingredients and how to use them alone, or in combinations, to treat the many common maladies that do not require a doctor's visit.

What About Problems with Over-the-Counter Drugs and Self-Care?

As in most other facets of life, there is good news and bad news. The downside of over-the-counter drugs must be recognized and kept in mind when choosing the self-care alternative. If the over-the-counter product does not work, for example, the potential savings in time, money, and reduced suffering are lost, and effective treatment is delayed. For this reason, the recommendations in this book are for the best agent at the optimal dose. An ineffective dose is even worse than not taking the drug at all because a risk of side effects or toxicity (albeit a small one) is taken, but no benefit can be expected.

Use of over-the-counter drugs may delay a visit to the doctor, and if the illness turns out to be serious instead of minor, significant additional illness or damage to your health may result. For this reason, you must carefully consider your symptoms and overall health status, and not ignore label instructions regarding how long to self-treat, or when to consult a physician for a given problem.

False claims and fringe products in the over-the-counter market erode the confidence of the public and produce many problems by causing people to give up self-treatment, and thereby suffer needlessly when effective products are available. Many professionals instill fear of damaging your health by self-care with over-the-counter drugs. In fact, problems related to self-medication are quite rare, indicating that people do exercise good judgment and make appropriate choices when self-care is selected.

A significant problem with over-the-counter drugs is the confusion generated by the marketing ploys of many companies. The names and ingredients of products are often very confusing. The same brand name may be used for products with very different ingredients; the same ingredient may be used under many different brand names. Often a code letter or number or other modifying word is used to distinguish one product from another product that contains different ingredients. This is done to capitalize on brand name recognition by the public. Also, over the years and especially recently, the formulation of many products has been changed to remove inactive or unsafe ingredients (as mandated by the USFDA). In some cases the product has been completely changed, while retaining a "brand name" that consumers recognize and accept. Be sure to read the ingredients listed on the label (they are required by law to be listed), and the amounts of each, to see if you are getting the medicine you want at the appropriate dose.

Perhaps the biggest problems with over-the-counter drugs are the lack of education provided to consumers and the overuse of combination drugs. Many manufacturers combine four to six or more drugs in a product in order to make grandiose claims of covering all the imaginable symptoms with a single product, needlessly exposing people to numerous drugs and possible drug interactions or side effects. Often a single drug or two drugs would suffice (and be cheaper). Much of the opposition from health professionals to over-the-counter drugs is leveled at this one issue. This book summarizes the individual ingredients, their use and benefits, as well as the combination drugs, and makes recommendations that allow the optimal use of both single ingredients and combinations, depending on the consumer's preferences, needs, and desires.

Use of Over-the-Counter Drugs by Special Populations

The use of over-the-counter products by children and seniors is safe and effective when label directions are carefully followed. The treatment of children is especially difficult, since they have limited experience with judging the nature and severity of their symptoms and the degree of relief afforded by treatment. Many of the over-the-counter drugs have been formulated especially for children, with adjusted doses. The drugs are also easier to administer and more palatable (flavored, liquids, and so on). Many over-the-counter drugs do not include doses for children under 12 years of age. This is because the USFDA requires that the drugs be tested in each specific age-group population, and the drug must be shown safe and effective in each group. Many companies do not perform these tests due to the expense and difficulties involved. This does not mean the drugs cannot be used. In many cases the label instructs you to consult your doctor. In this case the doctor assumes the liability for recommending the dose.

Children are not small adults. There are many changes that occur in the body as it grows and matures. Especially children under two are rapidly changing. In most cases, the appropriate dose must be based on a combination of factors including age, size, and even body surface area, to take into account all of the variables. With over-the-counter drugs, the margin of safety is greater than for prescription drugs, so the weight or age can generally be used to calculate the appropriate dose and be within the safe and effective level for the drug. The first thing to do is look on the label to see if dosages for children are given. Generally, you can calculate a dose by assuming that an adult weighs 120 pounds and the child is some fraction of that. For example, a 40-pound child would take one-third the adult dose. If the child has any preexisting disease, then all bets are off, and a physician should be consulted for determination of the appropriate dose. Follow label directions carefully in determining both the dose and frequency of use.

Numerous studies have shown that the elderly are the heaviest users of over-the-counter drugs. They are the segment of the population that has the highest incidence of illness. They also have the most experience with symptoms and self-treatment, but their bodies are also changing with age, and the tolerance for drugs and their ability to eliminate the drugs normally may be impaired.

The predictability of drug effects in seniors is less certain than in the younger population. In general, lower doses are equally effective due to multiple changes in the body that reduce the elimination of drugs and increase their effectiveness. This makes seniors more susceptible to the adverse side effects of all drugs. Concurrent use of other drugs, especially prescription drugs, will often alter the response to over-the-counter drugs and vice versa. This is a very complicated situation and must be individualized for the patient and the drugs used, in order to appropriately treat the ailment(s). Where available, such possible interactions and warnings are indicated.

Pregnant women are the hardest of all segments of the population to treat safely, since very little is known about the possibility of rare but serious effects that drugs may have on a developing baby. In general, drugs should be avoided during pregnancy. When treatment is necessary, the selection should be heavily influenced by the accumulated experience with the drug, sticking to widely used, time-proven drugs where no indication of problems have been noted. Such treatment should be discussed with your doctor.

Nursing mothers must also be very careful about the use of over-the-counter drugs. Many drugs taken by the mother appear in the breast milk and some may even be concentrated into the milk. The baby then gets a dose of the drug similar to or perhaps higher than the mother's. Where known, this information is included for the drugs recommended in this book. Always consider the distinct possibility that the baby will be getting any drug that a nursing mother takes.

The Placebo Effect and Over-the-Counter Drugs

The placebo effect is the benefit that results when a "sugar pill" (a pill with no medicinal value) is found to provide relief or benefit to some patients. Although some of this benefit is simply due to natural healing or resolution of the illness or symptom, the mind also has powerful effects on the body and on the perception of symptoms. It is clear that giving a pill, even one that cannot have any direct medical effects, is effective for a proportion of those treated.

For this reason, to prove that a drug is truly effective, it must be tested in comparison to a placebo. This must be done without the knowledge of the patient or observer (doctor, nurse, or other health-care professional) since knowing a pill is a placebo reduces its effectiveness. Most drugs, both over the counter and prescription, have been shown to have significant benefit through this type of study. It is not "tricking" the body, but somehow the placebo effect actually stimulates well-being.

This effect should not be taken lightly. In most studies, symptoms in 20% to 40% of patients are reduced by placebo treatment. Drug treatment must produce significantly better results (example: 50% to 80% of patients made better by active drug) in order to conclude that the drug is truly useful for the symptom or illness. What this means is that often half of the patients who benefit from treatment are made better by the placebo effect and the other half by the actual drug effect. Of course this varies depending on the drug, but it is an important part of the effectiveness of nearly all drugs. Since this effect occurs regardless of the drug, it is best to use the safest drug first to avoid possible problems while expecting good effects. This is a good argument for trying over-the-counter drugs before resorting to the more toxic, prescription-only drugs.

Health Care in the United States

Medical practices in the United States are quite different from those in many other countries. We spend more on health care than any other nation, yet we do not have the healthiest population, partly because our care is so expensive and not available to all. Americans are unusually aggressive and impatient for health care, forcing doctors to treat us when those in many other countries would not.

We rarely die of "natural causes"; there is always a disease that is the cause of our passing. We tend to view things as absolutes. For example, things like salt, fat, and cholesterol are viewed as unmitigated evils. Each of these is essential to life and good health and, in fact, each must be in a "middle range" to maintain optimal health. We tend to go to extremes, thinking the lowest cholesterol, or the lowest blood pressure, and so on, is most desirable.

We treat early, we treat aggressively, and we cause much illness with our overuse of drugs. Many illnesses are self-limiting (they go away spontaneously after running their course) and are not amenable to any treatment, except for symptomatic relief. Doctors are particularly guilty, as studies show that many prescriptions are written needlessly in response to real or perceived pressure from patients. Reasons cited most often for inappropriate or unnecessary drug prescribing are: (1) patient demand, (2) the intentional use of the placebo effect, and (3) a doctor's "personal experience" that convinces him or her that a drug is effective for a certain indication when objective, scientific testing has shown it is not.

How Drugs Work

Each and every drug works somewhat differently; however, there are many properties shared by all drugs. There are recognized "rules" of how drugs are able to accomplish what they do. First, drugs act either by being applied topically, directly to the site where the effect is desired (sprayed, rubbed, soaked, and so on); or they are taken systemically (by mouth, injection, suppository, and so on) so that the drug enters the bloodstream and is distributed and circulated throughout the body. Local effects and the number of drugs working this way are limited, and this book describes how they are used and which indications can be treated this way in detail.

Most drugs, even when given by different routes, end up in the blood and are carried to all parts of the body. Many have effects both at the local site and on remote areas, which contribute to the overall benefit. All drugs have a limited duration of effect and must be taken repeatedly to have persistent effects. The time between doses or the frequency with which each drug must be taken varies because drugs are handled differently by the body. Some drugs are eliminated by the kidneys, which filter or extract the drug from the blood and deposit it in the urine. This can be very rapid or quite slow. Other drugs are changed or eliminated by the liver or lungs into what are called metabolites, which are often inactive, but which may also have effects that contribute to the overall drug effect. Several other organs may also help to change or eliminate drugs from the body.

Ultimately, all drugs are made inactive and/or removed from the body to terminate their effects. Usually this happens within just a few hours. Since most drugs must be present—and present at a high enough concentration to have certain effects to be beneficial—repeated doses are needed. A greater effect is usually achieved by increasing the dose, but it is important to recognize that there is an upper limit to every drug's effect, and higher doses do not always yield a better effect. After a drug is taken, the effect comes on gradually as the drug enters the blood and the concentration increases. Then elimination starts and the level begins to fall.

With both absorption and elimination constantly going on, the drug level also changes constantly. What is desired is that the effective level of the drug be maintained over a reasonably narrow range that works but which does not produce undesirable or toxic effects. By taking larger doses, or especially by not taking the drug at the prescribed frequency (number of times a day or correct number of hours between doses), the level of the drug exceeds the desired level, or fluctuates between much higher and lower levels than are optimal. For this reason, it is much better to take the drug as indicated (dose and timing) for the best effect. If you are above average in size or more resistant to a drug, increasing the frequency of doses (shortening the time between doses) is more effective than taking a higher dose than is recommended.

How to Use This Book

This book is divided into chapters addressing each of the major body systems and/or the major symptoms to be treated. In the Contents, you can find the chapter that covers the topic you are interested in and turn to that page. For a specific symptom or illness you can also refer to the **Subject and Ingredients Index** (page 231) to locate the information. Each chapter contains sections devoted to specific disorders or treatments. For each topic, the details of symptoms, indications for drug use, and information about how symptoms are treated is explained. Each of these indications is followed by the recommendations for the best over-the-counter drugs to be used. Finally, examples of various brands containing the ingredient(s) are listed for reference.

If you have a brand name product and want to know how it is rated, refer to the **Brand Name Index** (pages 219–230). If a product is not listed by name, look up the active ingredient in the **Subject and Ingredient Index** (pages 231–234). This will refer you to the page or pages with a complete description of what it is for and how it ranks, along with information on appropriate uses. Chain store brands of the equivalent medicines are not listed because, without exception, they declined or did not respond to requests to make this information available. Some stated that they would not respond because their formulations changed from lot to lot based on where and who made the particular batch (lowest bidder contract work).

Finally, for fast reference to a particular symptom or illness, or to learn what a particular ingredient is primarily used for, refer to the **Quick-Reference Chart** located just after the Contents at the beginning of the book. This chart lists the most widely used ingredients and the most common symptoms with the page numbers where information is found in the book.

2

Pain and Fever— Internal Care

Analgesics are drugs that relieve pain, and antipyretics reduce fever. These two effects are common to a number of drugs, three of which are recommended for self-care. We consume thousands of pounds of these drugs each year as single entities or in combination products. *Aspirin* is the cheapest and best known of these agents, followed by acetaminophen, which has fewer side effects than aspirin, but is also less effective. *Acetaminophen* also lacks the important anti-inflammatory activity of aspirin, making it generally less desirable overall. The best drug in this class is *ibuprofen*, which was switched from prescription-only to over-the-counter availability several years ago. Ibuprofen is the most effective drug in this class for reducing pain and fever, and it has potent anti-inflammatory effects that add to its value for treating many of the indications noted. It also has fewer side effects than aspirin. A fourth drug just recently approved, *naproxen sodium,* is similar to ibuprofen except that its effect lasts longer, so doses are taken less frequently. However, this convenience, plus the lack of generic versions, makes it quite a bit more expensive than the other drugs. For this reason it is not recommended; but if you want the convenience and are willing to pay for it, just consider it a longer lasting version of ibuprofen.

General Pain and Fever Reducers

Each of these analgesics/antipyretics is usually taken orally, but the pain-relieving activity is effective throughout the body. A combination of local and central (brain) effects counteracts the pain and reduces the perception of pain. These drugs can also be given by suppository (into the rectum) if the patient is unable to take the medicine by mouth (for example, if vomiting occurs), although this is a less common route of administration.

Another method of pain relief is topical application of drugs known as local anesthetics. These drugs block the transmission of pain messages to the brain by acting locally on the sensors of pain or their nerves. The indications where this method is particularly effective are described, and suggestions are given for the best products in this class.

A combination of local (topical) and oral products achieve maximum pain relief. In virtually all cases, the oral route generally has the more pronounced overall effect and should not be overlooked (even for toothache, sunburn, and so on, where you might think the local treatment would be better).

All of these medications come in numerous physical forms, including pills, capsules, drops, elixirs, chewable tablets, liquids, gums, gelcaps, and enteric coated tablets. They are also frequently combined with buffers (to reduce stomach upset), flavorings, or with other active ingredients for special indications. Special forms are manufactured for children's and infants' use and to make them easier to swallow or to taste better. Extra-strength forms give you a higher than normal dose of the drug or combine two or more ingredients (or add caffeine) to provide extra pain relief.

This chapter makes specific recommendations for the use of these analgesics/antipyretics. It covers numerous indications and special considerations for different individuals, including senior citizens, adults, children, and infants and gives suggested doses. In all cases, the manufacturer's instructions supersede those given here, because the product may contain additional ingredients that limit the dose in some way. The dose listed here is the optimal dose for producing the maximum desired effect when the drug is used alone.

Generic names are always used, and some brand names are listed as examples for further reference. Always compare the active ingredient(s) and dose(s) of the product you intend to purchase with those recommended to be sure that you are getting the best drug and the optimal dose when you take the product according to the instructions on the label.

Active Ingredients for Pain and Fever

There are four major, active ingredients in this class to choose from, but there are literally thousands of products available that contain them, either as the ingredient alone or in combination with other ingredients. There are many different forms. Which you use is really a matter of personal preference and how much you are willing to pay.

Buy the generic (active ingredient name) or a house brand from a major chain store for the best price, or a name brand if you prefer. There are no real differences in safety or effectiveness when the active ingredient and dose are the same. Flavorings, buffers, and special formulations (gum, enteric coated, gelcaps, and so on) usually increase the cost but have limited practical usefulness. However, they are not ineffective, they just cost more.

Acetaminophen. Acetaminophen is an analgesic/antipyretic that is useful for mild pain and fever reduction. It is particularly good for children. It does not cause stomach upset or bleeding (aspirin does). Used for over 35 years, toxic effects are unusual when label instructions are followed, but an overdose can cause serious kidney or liver damage. **Pregnant women:** safety not established, but routinely used with no evidence of adverse effects. **Nursing mothers:** no evidence of risk, but it is secreted into the breast milk in low concentrations. **Seniors:** no special problems. **Drug interactions:** alcohol—heavy drinking increases risk of liver damage.

Aspirin. Aspirin has been used for over 90 years. It reduces pain and fever and has other useful effects, including reducing inflammation and preventing blood clots. It is present in many combination drugs for colds, menstrual discomfort, and other ailments. It tends to irritate the stomach and even may cause bleeding (ulcers). A rare brain and liver disease (Reye's syndrome) has occurred in children and young adults taking aspirin during viral infections. Aspirin is used so frequently, and often in doses exceeding what is recommended, that it accounts for more overdose/toxic reactions than any other drug. **Pregnant women:** not usually recommended, but frequently used. Its use should be restricted due to possible effects on the fetus. **Nursing mothers:** appears in breast milk. **Seniors:** no special problems. **Drug interactions:** alcohol—increased risk of stomach irritation and ulcers; anticoagulants—altered blood clotting time; steroids—increased stomach irritation.

Ibuprofen. Ibuprofen is a potent analgesic/antipyretic with pronounced anti-inflammatory activity. It relieves mild to moderate pain of all kinds and only rarely causes stomach upset or bleeding. In use for over 25 years, it is overall one of the best drugs switched from prescription-only to over-the-counter use. It is the overall best choice in this class. **Pregnant women:** not usually recommended; may cause problems, but no evidence of risk. **Nursing mothers:** no evidence of risk to infant. **Seniors:** reduced dose desirable or increased side effects may occur. **Drug interactions:** antidiabetic agents—decreased effects are noted; antihypertensive and diuretic drugs—reduced effects seen; anticoagulants, steroids, and alcohol—increased stomach irritation.

Naproxen sodium. This is the most recent drug to be changed from prescription-only to over-the-counter availability. Very similar to ibuprofen in nearly all respects, the only differences are that it lasts longer and it may have a slightly increased incidence of stomach upset. You don't need to take it as often to have continued effects or to maintain the optimal level of drug in your system. It is effective and particularly useful for arthritis because of its anti-inflammatory effects. Since it is only available in one brand (Aleve) and it is longer lasting, it costs considerably more than ibuprofen. **Pregnant women:** not usually recommended; may cause problems, but no evidence of risk. **Nursing mothers:** no evidence of risk to infant. **Seniors:** reduced dose desirable or increased side effects may occur. **Drug interactions:** antidiabetic agents—decreased effects are noted; antihypertensive and diuretic drugs—reduced effects seen; anticoagulants, steroids, and alcohol—increased stomach irritation.

Caffeine. Caffeine is a naturally occurring drug found in several plants and used very widely for its stimulatory effects. It is not an analgesic or antipyretic but is used to enhance the effect of analgesics. Most cultures have traditional beverages containing caffeine, which are heavily used. It stimulates the central nervous system and usually produces decreased drowsiness, less fatigue, and a more rapid and clear flow of thought. It can also enhance concentration and reflex time. Additional effects of this drug include stimulation of water loss by effects on the kidney, stimulation of the heart muscle, and relaxation of smooth muscle. Caffeine has been shown to enhance the pain relieving effects of most analgesics and is frequently combined with them in pain relief products. It may also be used to counteract the drowsiness-inducing potential of other drugs, especially antihistamines. **Pregnant women:** crosses placenta, but no evidence of risk. **Nursing mothers:** passes into the breast milk. **Seniors:** use with caution in the presence of heart disease, kidney disease, or concurrent use of psychological drugs. **Drug interactions:** heart drugs, psychological drugs—use with caution.

General Pain Relief and Fever Reduction (Oral Use)

FIRST CHOICE *for seniors, adults, children*

Generic name: Ibuprofen
Dose: 200–400 mg/dose
Maximum: 2,400 mg/day

Brand names: Addaprin, Advil, Arthritis Foundation Ibuprofen, Bayer Select Pain Relief, Genpril, Haltran, Medipren, Motrin IB, Nuprin, Ultraprin, Valprin

Reasons: Although ibuprofen is somewhat more expensive than aspirin or acetaminophen, it is the most effective analgesic and is safer to use than aspirin. It provides pain relief and fever reduction and counters inflammation. Take it with meals to reduce stomach upset (if it occurs). Ibuprofen slowly enters the joints and stays longer, so is very good for therapy of chronic arthritis.

Cautions: Ibuprofen may cause stomach upset (nausea or vomiting) and rarely can cause ulcers (much less than aspirin). Diarrhea or constipation may occur in some people. It is not recommended for pregnant or breast-feeding women, but there is no evidence of risk to the infant. Patients with kidney disease should consult a doctor before using these products. Ibuprofen may interact with antihypertensive (blood pressure) drugs, diuretics (water pills), alcohol, antacids, and anticoagulants. Consult your doctor if you take these medications. **Seniors:** a reduced dose may be desirable for seniors.

General Pain Relief and Fever Reduction (Oral Use)

FIRST CHOICE *for infants (under five years old)*

Generic name: Acetaminophen

Dose: Liquid 24–100 mg/ml; tablets 24–80 mg/tablet. Dose depends on the age and size of the infant. See label for instructions.

Brand names: Acetaminophen drops, Anacin-3 Infant's drops, Dorcol Children's Non-aspirin Fever and Pain Reducer, Genapap Children's Elixir, Halenol Children's Liquid, Liquiprin (Elixir and solution), Oraphen-PD, Panadol Children's (chewable and liquid), St. Joseph Aspirin-Free (drops and liquid), Tylenol (tablets, drops, elixir)

Reasons: Acetaminophen is the best choice for infants, due primarily to limited experience in this age group with ibuprofen. It is the gentlest of the three analgesic drugs, which also makes it the choice for all ages if stomach upset or susceptibility to ulcers is a problem.

Cautions: Overdoses of acetaminophen most often have toxic effects on the liver and this drug should not be used by individuals with a history of heavy alcohol use or with any liver disease. Its safety in pregnancy has not been established, but it is routinely used with no evidence of side effects. For nursing mothers there is no evidence of risk to the infant, but low concentrations of drug are found in breast milk. It can interact with alcohol, anticoagulants (blood thinners), and with food, and should not be taken simultaneously with these agents.

General Pain Relief and Fever Reduction (Oral Use)

SECOND CHOICE *for seniors, adults*

THIRD CHOICE *for children (over five years old)*

Generic name: Aspirin

Dose: 325–850 mg/dose

Maximum: 4,000 mg/day

Brand names: Anacin, Arthritis Foundation Safety Coated Asprin, Bayer Aspirin, Ecotrin, Empirin, Norwich Aspirin, St. Joseph Aspirin

Reasons: Aspirin is the standard for pain relief and fever reduction. It is also very inexpensive and is anti-inflammatory. More stomach upset (nausea and vomiting) and a higher potential for causing ulcers than ibuprofen makes it less desirable overall. Risks of overdose are also more significant with aspirin.

Cautions: Thousands of cases of overdose with aspirin occur each year because people do not respect this drug for what it really is, a potent, effective drug with significant toxicity. People take it in larger doses and more frequently than they should. Heavy use will induce significant damage to the stomach lining (ulcers) and may also result in nutrient depletion (especially iron). It interacts with antidiabetic drugs and anticoagulants (blood thinners). It is not usually recommended for pregnant women, but is frequently used. Its use should be restricted. Nursing mothers should be aware that aspirin passes into the breast milk.

General Pain Relief and Fever Reduction (Oral Use)

SECOND CHOICE *for children (over five years old)*

THIRD CHOICE *for seniors, adults*

Generic name: Acetaminophen

Dose: 325–1,000 mg / dose

Maximum: 4,000 mg/day

Brand names: Acetaminophen, Aminofen, Anacin-3, Arthritis Foundation Aspirin-Free, Arthritis Pain Formula-Aspirin-Free, Datril, Excedrin, Halenol, Panadol, Phenaphen, Tylenol, Valadol

Reasons: Acetaminophen is the second choice for children (ibuprofen is first choice) due to the rare occurrence of Reye's syndrome when aspirin (the third choice) is given to children who have viral infections.

Cautions: Acetaminophen can cause liver damage when taken in large quantities or over long periods of time. It interacts with alcohol, anticoagulants, and food. Safety is not established for pregnant women and nursing mothers, but it is widely used and appears to be safe.

Buffers and Special Formulations

Buffers reduce the stomach upset commonly caused by analgesic agents, and help reduce the irritation and ulcer-forming effects particularly prevalent with aspirin. Other special formulations are used to make the drugs easier to take (for example, liquids, coated tablets, flavorings, and sweeteners to make the taste more acceptable). Extra-strength formulations may contain a higher dose of the drug, a combination of two or more of the drugs, or caffeine to enhance the drug's effectiveness. All of these measures do have reasonable arguments and data to support their benefit. However, the benefit is often small compared to the significant increase in cost often seen for these products. This section lists some of the various special formulations and recommendations for their use.

Buffered and Special Formulations

FIRST CHOICE

Generic name: Ibuprofen

Dose: 200–400 mg

Reasons: Only tablets and capsules containing ibuprofen are currently readily available. Watch for special formulations in the future if desired. Ibuprofen can be taken with food, which works well if stomach upset occurs. This is the main reason for adding buffers to the other agents of this class. Buffered ibuprofen is probably not necessary, due to the low incidence of stomach upset and possibility of bleeding with this drug. Caffeine may be added to ibuprofen to increase its pain relieving effects. However, if other forms of caffeine (coffee, colas, other medications) are concurrently used, not only will the possible benefit be blunted because of the routine use of caffeine, but the possibility of an overdose of caffeine increases dramatically.

Buffered and Special Formulations

SECOND CHOICE

Generic name: Aspirin

Buffered tablets and liquids: Alka-Seltzer, Alka-Seltzer Flavored Ascriptin, Buffaprin, Buffasal, Bufferin Tri Buffered, Buffinol, Magnaprin

Suppositories: ASA Suppositories, Aspirin Suppositories

Flavored, chewable: St. Joseph Low Dose

Gum: Aspergum

Enteric coated: Ecotrin, Ecotrin Maximum Strength

Timed Release: Bayer 8-Hour Timed Release, Measurin Timed Release

Extra-strength aspirin is available in the following forms and brand names.

Larger dose: Alka-Seltzer Extra Strength, Arthritis Pain Formula, Bayer Aspirin Maximum, Norwich Extra Strength, Stanback Max Powder

With caffeine: Anacin Maximum Strength, BC Tablet/ Powder Arthritis Strength, Cope, Gensan, Midol and Midol Maximum, PAC, Salabuff

With caffeine and acetaminophen: Analval, Buffets II, Duradyne, Excedrin Extra Strength, Goody's Extra Strength, Neogesic, Panodynes, Saleto, Supac, Tenol Plus, Trigesic, Tri-pain, Vanquish

Buffered (extra strength): Ascriptin Extra Strength, Bufferin Arthritis Strength, Cama Arthritis Pain Reliever

---

Buffered and Special Formulations

THIRD CHOICE

Generic name: Acetaminophen

Buffered tablets and liquid: Bromo Seltzer

Suppositories: Acephen, Acetaminophen Uniserts, Feverall Children's, Neopap, Suppap-120/325/650

Drops and liquids: Aceta, Anacin-3 Infant's Drops, Dorcol Children's Non-Aspirin, Myapap Drops, Oraphen-PD, Panadol Infants', St. Joseph Aspirin-Free, Tempra Drops, Tylenol Children's

Flavored, chewable: Anacin-3 Chewable, Apacet Chewable, Genapap Chewable, Panadol Children's, St. Joseph Aspirin-Free, Tempra Chewable, Tylenol Children's

Flavored, liquid: Genapap Children's Elixir/Drops, Halenol Children's, Liquiprin Children's, Panadol Children's, St. Joseph Aspirin-Free, Tempra Syrup, Tylenol Children's

Extra-strength acetaminophen is available in the following forms and brand names.

Larger dose: Anacin 3 Maximum, Arthritis Pain Formula Aspirin Free, Aspirin Free Pain Relief, Banesin, Dapa Extra Strength, Datril Extra Strength, Genapap Extra Strength, Genebs Extra Strength, Halenol Extra Strength, Meda Cap, Pain Eze, Panadol, Panex 500, Tapanol Extra Strength, Tylenol Extra Strength, Valorin Super

With caffeine: Bayer Select Headache

With caffeine and aspirin: Analval, Buffets II, Duradyne, Excedrin Extra Strength, Goody's Extra Strength, Neogesic, Panodynes, Rid-A-Pain, SAC, Salatin, Saleto, Supac, Tenol Plus, Trigesic, Tri-pain, Vanquish

Suppositories. Rectal administration of analgesics is helpful for individuals who experience vomiting or significant stomach upset, from oral agents. Only aspirin and acetaminophen are currently available in suppository form, but ibuprofen probably will be available in the near future. The recommendations here are the same as for the oral doses: Aspirin is better for seniors and adults (more effective, but also more toxic). Acetaminophen is better for infants and children (including all teenagers), especially if mumps or flu is being treated, because of the widely recognized but rare complication of Reye's syndrome, which can occur in children (including teenagers) when aspirin is used for treating these viral diseases.

Suppositories for Pain and Fever (Rectal Administration)

FIRST CHOICE *for adults and seniors*

Generic name: Aspirin

Dose: 325–650 mg/dose

Brand names: ASA Suppositories, Aspirin Suppositories

Reasons: Aspirin is the standard for pain relief and fever reduction. It is also anti-inflammatory and less expensive than ibuprofen. Ibuprofen would be the first choice, but is not currently available in suppository formulation.

Cautions: Do not take oral and suppository forms of aspirin together, since both routes of administration result in the drug being absorbed into the blood and distributed throughout the body. This practice will result in an overdose. Thousands of cases of overdose with aspirin occur each year because people do not respect this drug for what it really is, a potent, effective drug with significant toxicity. They take it in larger doses and more frequently than they should. If you take multiple drugs, check to see if two or more contain aspirin or other similar drugs. When added together they result in an overdose of aspirin and are very likely to produce toxic effects.

Suppositories for Pain and Fever (Rectal Administration)

FIRST CHOICE *for children and infants*

Generic name: Acetaminophen

Dose: 60–325 mg/dose

Brand names: Acephen suppositories, Acetaminophen suppositories, Acetaminophen Uniserts, Feverall Children's, Neopap, Suppap-120/325/650

Reasons: Acetaminophen is the best choice for infants. It is the gentlest of the three drugs, which also makes it the choice for all ages if side effects are a problem.

Cautions: Do not take oral and suppository forms of acetaminophen together, since both routes of administration result in the drug being absorbed into the blood and distributed throughout the body. This practice will result in an overdose. If you take multiple drugs, check to see if two or more contain acetaminophen or other similar drugs. When added together, they result in an overdose of acetaminophen, and are very likely to produce toxic effects.

Specific Indications for Use of Pain and Fever Reducers

ACHES AND PAINS. For general aches and pains, the oral administration of ibuprofen for all ages except infants is the best choice. The drug acts both locally (but gets there through the blood) and in the brain to reduce the pain, and also reduces the inflammation (the symptoms noted as redness, warmth, and swelling) that is common to many of the causes of these aches and pains. Aspirin and acetaminophen, as described earlier, are second and third choices, depending on age. Some of these drugs are also available in creams or lotions to be rubbed on the site. There is no evidence that this method of use is effective. The act of rubbing, and even the local effects of a soothing or cooling cream or lotion, may distract your attention and provide some relief, but the drugs are not effective when given this way. These rather expensive products have no analgesic effect on pain. (See page 31 for more details.)

ARTHRITIS. Arthritis (rheumatoid arthritis) is a chronic, diffuse inflammatory disease involving primarily the joints, which affects about 1% of the U.S. population. The cause is unknown, but the incidence is higher in women than men. Onset is frequently associated with some stressful situation, either physical or emotional. It is a common affliction of the elderly. The symptoms of arthritis (pain and stiffness) are handled very well by treatment with ibuprofen and related agents. Even prescription drugs are probably no more effective than ibuprofen, except when the more toxic "disease modifying drugs" are needed to slow the progression of disease. If you are not able to get relief, you can try aspirin as an alternative therapy, but it would be better to visit your doctor for a more complete workup and intensive therapy (higher doses with monitoring for adverse effects) if you do not get satisfactory results. Doctors also have alternative drugs that are more toxic and may affect the course of the disease (preventing progression or slowing it down), which is particularly important if you have progressively worsening symptoms. A large number of topically applied analgesic agents are available for use in arthritis. However, none of these has been shown to be effective as an analgesic (pain reliever). This is not to say they have no effect. The act of rubbing them in, as well as local cooling effects on the skin, can alter the perception of pain and provide some relief. Since these drugs don't do what they claim to do, they are not recommended. If you want topical relief, use a cream or lotion that has local soothing effects (like menthol) or that serves as a lubricant or skin softener to facilitate the massage. Don't waste your money on expensive products that contain a drug that can't work because it stays on the surface of the skin. (See page 31 for more details.)

BACKACHE. Backache is a common problem, occurring in about 5% of the population. Only the common cold disables more adults each year. To treat acute strains of the back (the cause of 90% of backaches), just follow the general instructions for pain and fever. There are no other prescription agents or drugs for the treatment of backache that are superior to ibuprofen, aspirin, or acetaminophen. Combination agents with a "special ingredient" to relieve these symptoms have not been shown to have any additional action and may not be safe. Exercises to strengthen back muscles can be very effective (82% of people respond to exercise) and should be the longer term treatment, supplemented by ibuprofen as needed. The best treatment is to take care of your back by losing excess weight, lifting properly, and avoiding sitting in the same position for long periods of time (move around every 15–20 minutes). When you are sitting maintain a good posture: legs together (not crossed), feet on floor, back straight, head held up, and arms resting. Get up every hour to stretch, sleep on a firm mattress, eat right, and exercise. Yes, all of these things affect your back. The exercises should be directed at your back through your abdomen (belly). By doing easy, slow sit-ups, you can strengthen your back and relieve backache. Additional activities usually recommended for helping the back include backstroke swimming, brisk walking, stair climbing, bike riding (stationary or actual), and cross-country ski machines.

BURNS. For simple burns where the skin is not broken, first apply cold water to reduce the burning sensation. Oral analgesics are probably more effective overall than topical agents, the first choice of which is ibuprofen. It should be taken as soon as possible to help reduce redness and pain. Prevention of pain is more effective than treatment once pain sets in, so the earlier the drug is taken the better. Topical anesthetics also provide additional relief. Their use and recommendations for the best products are discussed in Chapter 3, page 44.

COLDS. Colds are caused by more than 150 separate viruses, and there is no cure, nor are there proven effective preventive measures (including large doses of vitamin C) for this very common ailment. The best you can do is rest and drink plenty of liquids to prevent dehydration. Pain or fever reducers (ibuprofen is best) relieve many of the common symptoms, and for the other symptoms, decongestants, cough suppressants, and so on, will provide additional relief. See the special section on flu and colds in Chapter 4.

CRAMPS, MENSTRUAL. Ibuprofen is the best choice. See Chapter 9 for more details and options.

CRAMPS, MUSCLE. Muscle cramps can temporarily disable even the fittest of athletes. They are very unpredictable, and their cause is not well understood. Most authorities now think that dehydration of the muscle is a major cause of cramps. The terms cramps and spasms are often used interchangeably to refer to painful, sustained, involuntary muscle contractions. Sometimes massaging or stretching the muscle will cause cramps to disappear, but not always. Fatigue and overexertion may be predisposing factors. Drinking water is the best overall treatment, with small frequent sips being most effective to prevent cramps. Potassium deficiency may also play a role in causing cramps. Products made specifically for the treatment of muscle cramps, which have more than a pain relieving ingredient, have been found to be unsafe or no more effective than the analgesic alone. The best treatment for immediate relief is to take ibuprofen and exercise the muscle to get the cramp out. Ice may also be effective to help the muscle relax, except in cases where exposure to cold may have helped precipitate the cramp. In this case warming would be helpful.

EARACHE. Earache is a common complaint that may be used to describe a variety of symptoms. The source may be the ear itself, either the external or middle ear, as a result of infection. This must be treated with an antibiotic, available only by prescription from a doctor. However, dental pain and sinusitis may also cause apparent "earache." Even tonsillitis can cause ear or facial pain. Unfortunately, the locally applied remedies for earache have been found to be ineffective. The best way to handle an earache is to take the oral pain reliever, ibuprofen, or an alternative, as described earlier.

FEVER. Fever is a common symptom, which can be caused by many different diseases. It is a universal indicator that something is wrong and the body is fighting back, be it an infection or some malfunction of an organ. Ibuprofen is the best over-the-counter agent for reducing fever and helping other related symptoms, but it does not address the source of the problem nor cure the underlying disease. It only provides symptomatic relief. For viral infections like colds and flu that must run their normal course anyway, the symptom relief is useful. In other cases, taking pain relievers may only postpone seeking the proper treatment that cures the source of the fever (for example, a bacterial infection that must be treated with an antibiotic). Judgment and experience are the best guides to deciding when or whether or not to consult your doctor when you have a fever.

FLU (INFLUENZA). See the special section on colds and flu in Chapter 4.

HANGOVER. See Chapter 5, page 106.

HEADACHE. Everyone from time to time has headaches, and the causes are many. Severe headache may be a warning sign that something serious is wrong and appropriate medical treatment is required. Migraine, tension headache, and cluster headaches are not life-threatening, but they are major causes of morbidity (suffering and absence from work). Mild headaches are common, and have been so in nearly all societies for as long as time records. Ibuprofen is the best treatment for relief of simple headache pain. Caffeine, taken along with the pain reliever, provides more symptom relief than ibuprofen alone (or aspirin or acetaminophen). In some cases, combinations of two agents with or without caffeine are used. Whether this is an advantage or not is unclear, but the rule of thumb should be to keep the number of drugs used to a minimum. Single agents are preferred except when additional symptoms warrant the use of another active ingredient for another specific symptom requiring relief. Preventive therapy is better than abortive treatment, so medication should be taken as soon as you notice the headache. If the headache is located behind the eyes or temples, a vascular component is likely, and the sinus medications (analgesic plus decongestant) may be more effective (see Chapter 4, page 59). Caffeine may also be more effective as an added ingredient for these types of headaches, but since it disrupts sleep and rest, and because sleep is often an important factor in curing a headache, it should be used sparingly (if at all), and especially not at night.

HEMORRHOIDS. Temporary relief from acute pain and itching caused by hemorrhoids can be achieved by application of topical anesthetics as described in Chapter 3. In order to promote healing and reduce inflammation, other therapies, including topical preparations that include protectants to reduce irritation, are better. See the section on hemorrhoids in Chapter 3, beginning on page 46.

INGROWN TOENAILS. Little can be done to toughen the skin or make the nail grow out faster, or over the skin, without a visit to your doctor and a surgical solution (removing the nail or reducing its size). Temporary pain relief can be achieved with local anesthetics (see Chapter 3, page 46) or oral pain medication (see page 21). Although not a major or frequent problem, there is an additional small risk of adverse effects from an allergic reaction to the topical agents. For more information, see Chapter 6, page 111.

INSECT BITES/STINGS. A large number of insects bite or inflict painful stings, causing great discomfort and, in certain cases, resulting in life-threatening allergic reactions (anaphylaxis). For anyone who has had a serious reaction to such a sting, consultation with a physician is important so that preventive measures or self-administered life-saving treatment can be kept available. However, in the vast majority of cases, the sting or bite is only a temporary discomfort. Many folk remedies are touted for this problem, but none has been proven effective (including meat tenderizer). The best therapy is to provide pain relief with oral medication (page 21) and local relief using the local anesthetics (see Chapter 3, page 44) or skin soothing agents like calamine lotion (see Chapter 6, page 145).

MUSCLE ACHES. Use standard oral pain relievers for muscle aches. Special products that claim to be useful are no more effective than ibuprofen alone. The numerous topical analgesics really only provide local sensations that seem to reduce pain by their cooling effect or the effect of the massaging of the site in applying the preparation (by increasing the blood flow). Topical application of analgesics is not effective (not to be confused with local anesthetics, which will deaden surface pain, see Chapter 3, page 44). Local anesthetics cannot penetrate deeply enough to be effective for the muscles. Warmth and massage are effective and are good supplements for the oral analgesics ibuprofen, aspirin, or acetaminophen (see discussion starting on page 21).

OSTEOARTHRITIS. A frequent cause of physical impairment in the elderly, osteoarthritis has a slow, progressive course of deteriorating joints. More than 65% of Americans over the age of 65 have X-ray evidence of osteoarthritis, but only one-third to one-half have symptoms. The hands and main weight-bearing joints are most commonly affected, but animals, including swimming mammals that have no weight-bearing joints, also suffer from this disease. The cause of osteoarthritis is unknown, but trauma or other factors affecting the joints tend to precipitate development of this disease. Joint pain, tenderness, and stiffness are the major manifestations. It can occur at younger ages, with the feet, wrists, and spine being initial sites of onset with increasing age. Strangely, the ankle joint is rarely involved. The pain is usually poorly localized and initially occurs in episodes associated with activity. As with rheumatoid arthritis, osteoarthritis can be as effectively treated (the symptoms, not the cause) with ibuprofen (or over-the-counter drugs) as with prescription medicines. To help maintain joint function, strengthening and range of motion exercises are very useful. If over-the-counter drugs do not provide adequate relief, you should see your doctor for a complete workup and intensive therapy. Immobilization (lack of or reduced motion) is one of the worst things for osteoarthritis. Movement is beneficial, especially shorter, frequent periods of exercise. Heat applied to the affected joints is often helpful when applied before the activity; while cold applied after exercise can reduce discomfort and facilitate a shorter period of pain following the activity.

PILES. See Chapter 5, page 92, for treatment, or refer to "Hemorrhoids," above.

RECTAL ITCH. This is one of the few indications in this class of pain that is probably best treated by local application of products designed specifically for rectal itch, such as topical steroids. (See Chapter 3, page 45, for details.)

SORE THROAT. Specific and effective topical measures for sore throat are described in the next chapter. However, one of the most effective treatments to relieve the pain is the oral analgesic ibuprofen (or aspirin or acetaminophen) due to the way these drugs work and their effectiveness. Topical therapy is optimal using dyclonine, but other topical anesthetic agents are also effective.

SPRAINS AND STRAINS. What you do within the first 30 minutes after a sprain can make a big difference in how long your recovery will take. First, rest the sprain briefly, then check for broken bones. Just try to put a little weight on the site. Instinct should tell you in many cases whether or not it is broken (too painful to put weight on). If it feels numb or tingles or feels cold, it is best to see a doctor. Next, to help reduce the swelling, wrap it with an elastic bandage, with padding in the nooks and crannies to put pressure on the site. Alternate this pressure with ice as tolerated. Do not use heat. For the first 24 hours after a sprain, cold (ice packs) and oral ibuprofen provide the most relief and do the most good. After a day or two, warm, not hot, therapy (heating pad or soaks) and continued use of ibuprofen will provide the most relief. You should also start exercising by wiggling and moving the joint to limber it up and help it heal in a more "ordered" fashion. Continue to exercise, and increase it as tolerated to speed recovery and foster good healing.

SUNBURN. Oral pain relievers are the best treatment for sunburn, depending on the size of the skin area involved. If needed, supplement the pain relief therapy with topical anesthetics described in the next chapter (page 44). Drinking plenty of liquids helps to avoid other possible complications. Although not usually a major or frequent problem, there is a small risk of adverse effects from an allergic reaction to the topical agents. For more details and information, see Chapter 6, page 153.

TEETHING. It is difficult to evaluate the relief or lack thereof from drugs given to infants, but based on adult experiences and evaluation of anesthetic agents, the teething formulations are thought to be effective and helpful to some extent (see Chapter 3, page 42). Oral pain relief may be more useful overall (acetaminophen—see page 22), or the combination of oral and local pain relief can be used.

TOOTHACHE. Until the reason for the toothache is determined and treated, oral pain relievers (ibuprofen, aspirin, or acetaminophen) and local anesthetics may provide relief and some comfort. See the oral product suggestions (Chapter 3, page 21) and topical anesthetics (page 41) for local relief and treatment.

3

Pain—
External Care

In addition to, or instead of, the pain relieving drugs taken by mouth, there are quite a number of drugs for topical, or local, application to relieve the surface pain of burns, ingrown toenails, insect stings and bites, sore throat, teething, and toothache. Most of these products are sold for very specific purposes, but they commonly incorporate what are known as local anesthetics, which block pain signals transmitted to the brain. This chapter recommends the few that have been proven superior for the reasons stated. They fall into three categories: for use in the mouth, for use on the skin, and for use on mucous membranes. You may choose one that works for you, but if you don't try the suggested ones, you will probably not get the maximum relief, since many inferior agents are sold. In all cases, the oral pain relievers also work, and they provide additional, and usually superior, relief. Note that oral ibuprofen or aspirin are anti-inflammatory, but none of the local anesthetics is anti-inflammatory. Therefore, it is best to take the oral preparation and supplement it with the topical agent as needed for virtually all of the symptoms described.

Leading Local Anesthetics

Dyclonine. A local anesthetic with a rapid onset of effect and good absorption into the skin or mucous membranes, dyclonine is very safe (has a very low incidence of side effects). Allergic reactions are rare. Dyclonine is particularly well suited for topical oral use, for example in sore throat. **Pregnant women, nursing mothers, and seniors:** no reason to believe there are specific needs or problems for any special populations.

Benzocaine. Introduced 85 years ago, benzocaine is one of the first, and still one of the best, local anesthetics. It is used in many diverse formulations for relief of surface pain and itching. It is very poorly absorbed through the skin or mucous membranes, which makes it quite safe for general use. It has few adverse effects, although occasionally a person may become allergic. **Pregnant women, nursing mothers, and seniors:** no special problems.

Lidocaine. Lidocaine is a local anesthetic with a rapid onset of effect. It has more penetrating ability and a longer duration of effect (about one hour) than benzocaine and is widely available in different products for pain and itching. Used for over 40 years, it is quite safe and effective. **Pregnant women:** no evidence of risk. **Nursing mothers:** no evidence of risk, but do not apply to nipple. **Seniors:** no special problems.

Dibucaine. Dibucaine is a very potent local anesthetic with quite long-lasting effects. Due to these properties, it also has a higher incidence of side effects (headache and dizziness). Dibucaine is most useful for prolonged relief when the maximum anesthetic effect is desired and less frequent application is preferred. **Pregnant women:** no data. **Nursing mothers:** no data, but do not apply to nipple. **Seniors:** no data. (No reason to expect any problems.)

   Hydrocortisone. This drug is actually a hormone produced naturally by the body which belongs to another drug class (see Chapter 6). It is listed here as well because it is used topically to relieve itch and irritation due to its potent anti-inflammatory effects. It is used and is very effective in a wide variety of diseases and provides relief of several symptoms. Overuse may lead to permanent thinning of the skin as well as other more serious (but rare) adverse effects (altered mineral and fat metabolism). **Pregnant women:** no evidence of risk. **Nursing mothers:** may pass into milk. **Seniors:** no special problem, but a lower dose may be desirable to reduce the possibility of increasing thinning of the skin—a condition that already occurs normally in old age.

Other Local Anesthetics

There are a large number of other products available for use in this category, but they are not as effective or safe as those suggested. The following three drugs are widely used but provide incomplete local anesthetic affects:

- *Camphor* acts by stimulating a cold sensation on the skin or membranes to give the perception of relief without actually being an anesthetic (similar to putting ice on the site).

- *Menthol* is similar to camphor; it provides some relief, but is not the most effective agent in this class.

- *Phenol* also induces some numbness, but this effect is incomplete and is inferior to the recommended agents.

   An ever increasing number of analgesic agents, including aspirin, ibuprofen, acetaminophen, and others, are put in creams, ointments, or liquid form to be applied directly to the sore, aching, or painful site (muscles, joints, and so on). These agents either do not work or are at best poorly effective, especially considering what they cost. Although they usually contain active drugs, most of the drug is wasted (it just sits on the skin surface). Any benefit seems to come from the effects of rubbing the agent on the affected area, by increasing blood flow, and warming or cooling the site. They cost too much for what they are, therefore these agents are not recommended if you are seeking lasting, effective relief of pain or soreness. They will provide some local sensation (usually heating or cooling), and the placebo effect may be important as well; so if you find they work for you, go ahead and use them. Just keep in mind that the oral pain reliever, ibuprofen, is far more effective (see Chapter 2, page 21). Less expensive lotions, creams, and liquids will also work as well.

Brand Names Not Recommended. Absorbine Arthritic Pain, Absorbine Jr., Act-On Rub, Anabalm, Analgesic Balm, Argesic, Aspercreme, Banalg Muscle (or Arthritic) Pain Reliever, Bangesic, Baumodyne, Ben-Gay (multiple forms), Betuline, Counterpain Rub, Deep-Down, Dencorub, Dermal-Rub, Dermolin, Doan's Backache, Epi-derm, Exocaine, Flex-all 454, Foot Medic, Ger-O-Foam, Gordogesic, Heet, Icy Hot, Infra-Rub, Mentholatum Deep Heating, Minit-Rub, Mobisyl, Musterole Deep Strength, Myoflex, Omega Oil, Panalgesic Gold, Pronto, Rid-A-Pain, Sloan's, Soltice Quick Rub, Sportscreme, Stimurub, Surin, ThermoRub, Vicks VapoRub, Wonder Ice, Yager's Liniment

---

Sore Throat (Lozenges for Oral Use)

FIRST CHOICE *for seniors, adults, children*

Generic name: Dyclonine (HCl)

Adult dose: 3 mg

Pediatric dose: 1.2 mg

Brand names: Children's Sucrets Cherry Flavored, Sucrets Maximum Strength Sore Throat Lozenges

Reasons: Dyclonine is a very effective topical anesthetic, especially good for sore throat. It has very low toxicity, and can be used repeatedly (by lozenge) for temporary relief of sore throat.

Cautions: None of special concern.

Sore Throat (Lozenges for Oral Use)

SECOND CHOICE *for seniors, adults, children*

Generic name: Benzocaine

Dose: 5–32 mg

Brand names: Cepacol Troches, Chloraseptic Cool Mint, Soretts, Spec-T, Thorets, Vicks Throat Lozenges

Reasons: Benzocaine is the best overall general local anesthetic, useful for treating various types of local pain. Though dyclonine is the first choice for sore throat, benzocaine is also very effective and useful for this indication.

Cautions: Benzocaine has a somewhat increased incidence of side effects compared with dyclonine and a slight possibility of causing allergic reactions.

Toothache (Topical Use in the Mouth)

FIRST CHOICE *for seniors, adults, children*

Generic name: Benzocaine

Dose: 15–20 % conc.

Brand names: Anbesol Maximum Strength (gel and liquid), Benzodent, Dent's Dental Poultice, Orabase-B or O, Orajel

Reasons: Benzocaine is the best overall local anesthetic for topical use, having a good balance of effect, duration of action and safety. Some of the others are more potent or last longer, but have more toxicity, so products containing benzocaine are overall the best choice.

Cautions: Benzocaine has the lowest potential for side effects of all the alternatives for this treatment group.

Toothache (Topical Use in the Mouth)

SECOND CHOICE *for seniors, adults, children*

Generic name: Benzocaine

Dose: 5–10 % conc.

Brand names: Anbesol (gel and liquid), Jiffy Toothache Drops, Numzident Gel, Numzit Gel, Orajel and Oragel-D, Rid-A-Pain Gel, Tanac Liquid

Reasons: This is the same ingredient as the first choice, but in a lower dose. These products will not be as effective or long-lasting as the first choice products. However, they are recommended ober other ingredients for toothache.

Cautions: Benzocaine has the lowest potential for side effects of all the alternatives for this treatment group.

Teething

FIRST CHOICE *for infants*

Generic name: Benzocaine

Dose: 7.5 % conc.

Brand names: Baby Anbesol Gel, Baby Orajel, Numzit Gel

Reasons and cautions: Same as above for adult products.

Cold/Canker Sores and Fever Blisters (Topical Use Only— To Reduce Size of Sore)

FIRST CHOICE *for seniors, adults, children*

Generic names: Tannic acid *and* Salicylic acid

Dose: Tannic acid, 7% conc.; salicylic acid, 2.5% conc.

Brand names: Zilactol. Several other brands contain tannic acid with benzocaine, but it's not clear if they also reduce sore size. Examples are Orajel CSM, Orasept Liquid, Tannac (liquid, roll-on, and stick)

Reasons: Although the USFDA (U.S. Food and Drug Administration) has not yet ruled whether tannic acid is effective, a recent clinical trial showed a clear benefit in reducing the size of the sores when it was applied soon after the first symptoms were noted.

Cautions: These agents are safe, especially since they are used topically. They should not be ingested and should be applied directly on the sore to minimize irritating effects.

Cold/Canker Sores and Fever Blisters (Topical Use— Pain Relief Only)

SECOND CHOICE *for seniors, adults, children*

Generic name: Benzocaine

Dose: 15–20% conc.

Brand names: Anbesol Maximum Strength (gel and liquid), Benzodent, Kank-A Liquid Professional Strength, Orabase (B or O), Orajel Maximum Strength, Orajel Mouth Aid

Reasons: Benzocaine is the best overall local anesthetic for topical use, having a good balance of effect, duration, and safety. Some of the other drugs in this class are more potent or last longer, but have more toxicity; so products containing benzocaine are overall the best choice.

Cautions: Benzocaine has the lowest potential for side effects of all the alternatives for this treatment group.

Sunburn, Burns, Ingrown Toenail, Insect Bites/ Stings
(For Use on Unbroken Skin Only)

FIRST CHOICE *for seniors, adults, children*

Generic name: Benzocaine

Dose: 10–20 % conc.

Aerosols: aeroCaine, aeroTherm, Americaine, Burntame, Dermoplast, Lanacaine, Solarcaine, Tega Caine

Creams/lotions: Americaine, Benzocaine, Benzocol, Dermoplast, Foille, Lagol, Medicone Dressing, Solarcaine, Sting Kill (swabs), Sting Relief

Reasons: Benzocaine is the best overall local anesthetic for topical use, having a good balance of effect, duration, and safety. Some of the other drugs in this class are more potent or longer lasting, but they also have more toxicity associated with their use.

Cautions: Benzocaine has the lowest potential for side effects of all the alternatives for this treatment group.

Sunburn, Burns, Ingrown Toenail, Insect Bites/Stings
(For Use on Unbroken Skin Only)

SECOND CHOICE *for seniors, adults, children*

Generic name: Lidocaine *or* dibucaine

Dose: Lidocaine, 1–2.5 % conc.; dibuacaine, 1 % conc.

Brand names: After Burn Plus, Bactine First Aid, Dibucaine, Medi-Quik, Nupercainal Ointment, Unguentine Plus, Xylocaine

Reasons: These two alternatives for local anesthetic effect are both more potent and longer lasting than the first choice (benzocaine). However, they seem to be somewhat less effective overall, and have more toxic potential than benzocaine, so they remain the second choice.

Cautions: Due to possible side effects, follow label directions regarding the amount and timing of reapplication. If skin irritation occurs, discontinue use immediately.

Anal/Vaginal Itch (Mucous Membrane Use, for Relief of Itching)

FIRST CHOICE *for seniors, adults, children*

Generic names: Benzocaine *or* dibucaine

Dose: Benzocaine, 20% conc.; dibucaine, 1% conc.

Brand names: Americaine Ointment, Lanacane aerosol, Nupercainal ointment

Reasons: These drugs are widely used for treatment of localized pain and itching. Detailed descriptions for use are discussed on page 46 and in Chapter 9, 188. Also, see the recommendations below for the anti-inflammatory first choice agent that is good for relief of itching.

Anal/Vaginal Itch (For Anti-Inflammatory Effects, Topical Use)

FIRST CHOICE *for seniors, adults, children*

Generic name: Hydrocortisone

Dose: 1/2–1 % conc.

Brand names: Anusol HC-1, Bactine, CaldeCORT, Cortaid, Cortef Feminine Itch Cream, Cortizone-5, Cortisone-10, Delacort, Dermacort, Dermolate, Dermtex HC, FoilleCort, Gynecort Creme, H2Cort, Hydrocortisone, Hydro-Tex, Hytone, Lanacort, Pharmacort, Preparation HC, Racet SE, Rhulicort

Reasons: Hydrocortisone is a natural hormone that is used for a number of symptoms. It is a potent anti-inflammatory agent, which can reduce swelling, redness, and itching. It does not act very quickly, and the best effects are noted only after several days of use.

   Cautions: Overuse of this drug can result in permanent thinning of the skin and may allow infections to develop in wounds (broken skin) that would otherwise not occur. If large surfaces of the body are treated, general side effects (altered mineral and salt metabolism) can occur. Follow label directions for best results.

Specific Indications for Local Anesthetics

BURNS.   For simple burns where the skin is not broken, first apply cold water. Oral analgesics (first choice ibuprofen, as discussed in Chapter 2, page 21) should also be taken as soon as possible to help reduce redness and pain. Prevention of pain is more effective than treatment once pain sets in, so the earlier the drug is taken the better. Topical agents can be used exclusively, but are probably better used as supplements to oral pain and inflammation reducers (see pages 44 and 161).

COLD/CANKER SORES.   These sores on the lips or in the mouth are caused by viruses and are a recurring problem in 20–45% of the general population. Pain and discomfort are the most common symptoms, but they are usually resolved, or at least decreased, within a day or two. Therefore the treatment course is to relieve the symptoms. The size of the lesion may be reduced, and the pain can be lessened by the very early application of the topical treatment described on page 42. As soon as the earliest signs of a developing sore are noted, the medication should be applied. For relief of pain for an established sore, the second choice agents are topical anesthetics (see page 43).

HEMORRHOIDS.   Temporary relief from pain and itching caused by hemorrhoids can be achieved by application of topical anesthetics, but in order to promote healing and reduce inflammation, other preparations that include protectants to reduce irritation are better. See Chapter 5, page 92.

INGROWN TOENAILS.   Little can be done to toughen the skin or make the nail grow out faster, or over the skin, without a visit to your doctor and a surgical solution (such as removing the nail or reducing its size). Temporary pain relief can be achieved with the local anesthetics (page 44) or by oral pain medication (Chapter 2, page 38).

INSECT BITES/STINGS. Many folk remedies are touted for this problem, but none has been proven effective (including meat tenderizer). The most effective approach is to provide pain relief by giving oral medication (Chapter 2, page 21) and to provide topical relief using the local anesthetics (page 44), or skin-soothing agents (Chapter 6, page 160). A large number of insects bite or inflict stings, causing great discomfort and, in certain cases, resulting in life-threatening allergic reactions. For anyone who has had a serious reaction to such a sting, consultation with a physician is important so that preventive measures or self-administered life-saving treatment can be kept available. However, in the vast majority of cases, the sting or bite is only a temporary discomfort.

PILES. See "Hemorrhoids" (above) or Chapter 5, page 92.

RECTAL ITCH. For itching due to minor irritation, two choices are available. For simple relief of the itching, a locally applied topical anesthetic is the fastest and most effective (see page 45). If treatment for inflammation is desired, the best choice is a topical steroid cream (1% hydrocortisone cream), which is also described on page 45.

SORE THROAT. The best treatment to reduce sore throat pain is the local anesthetic, dyclonine, a topically effective and quite safe anesthetic especially suited to this use. Since it is available in only one major product, other alternatives have also been suggested (see use of local anesthetics, page 39).

SUNBURN. For sunburn, depending on the size of skin area involved, the best treatment is to take oral pain relievers (ibuprofen, see Chapter 2, page 21). If needed, apply the topical anesthetics described in this chapter to supplement pain therapy (page 44). Although not usually a major or frequent problem, there is a risk of adverse effects from an allergic reaction to the topical agents. This is not usually a major or frequent problem. For more details and information, see Chapter 6, page 161.

TEETHING. It is difficult to evaluate the relief, or lack thereof, from drugs given to infants, but, based on adult experiences and evaluation of anesthetic agents, the teething formulations are thought to be effective and helpful to some extent (see page 42). Oral pain relief may be more useful overall (acetaminophen, Chapter 2, page 19), or the combination of oral and local pain relief can be used.

TOOTHACHE. Until the reason for the toothache is determined and treated, oral pain relievers and topical anesthetics may provide relief and some comfort. See the product suggestions on page 41. For oral analgesic relief use ibuprofen (Chapter 2, page 20).

4

Respiratory System

This chapter deals with drugs that benefit respiratory functions and the symptoms of colds, flu, allergies, hay fever, and asthma. Three major groups of symptoms are covered:

- Colds and flu

- Allergies
- Asthma (wheezing)

None of the drugs cures the problems, but they provide relief of symptoms. For this reason the individual symptoms and the appropriate drugs and/or combinations, and treatment with single or combination products, are discussed. Both oral and topical agents are available and useful for many respiratory symptoms. Many people go to the doctor for treatment of colds or flu, but there is no curative treatment. These viral diseases must run their course, and recovery is due to the natural defenses of the body overcoming the virus. Over-the-counter medications can reduce symptoms. Only in some severe cases may hospitalization be required to handle serious symptoms or complications.

Respiratory illnesses are treated with several different classes of drugs, including cough suppressants, decongestants, antihistamines, expectorants, and bronchodilators. Each of the drugs alone, as well as each of these in combination with others, or with pain and fever reducers (see Chapter 2, pages 21–24), will be discussed and recommendations made. This is a very complicated group of products to recommend. Several hundred are available, and there is a bewildering array of possible combinations that result when multiple classes of drugs are combined. Useful comparisons are very difficult to make. Especially in this class, many of the products contain alcohol as an additional ingredient (see Chapter 8, page 172). Alcohol can produce additional effects that may be desirable or undesirable, depending on the individual and circumstances (time of day, need to function effectively at work, desire for sleep, and so on).

Colds and Flu

The next several sections sort out the symptoms of colds and flu individually and recommend the optimal treatment for each symptom. It is always best not to take more drugs than are necessary to treat the symptoms you are experiencing. Symptoms and severity vary from person to person. Since some of the drugs may cause drowsiness or excitability, you can reduce side effects by taking only the drugs warranted for your particular symptoms. When combination agents are used, it is sometimes a real challenge to find one that combines the best agent in each category, so it may be better to have each individual agent and take each one as needed rather than follow the "shotgun" approach of taking one pill or liquid preparation with everything thrown into it.

There are many myths about colds and flu. Some people claim that bathing or showering in the morning reduces your resistance to colds or flu. Many people insist that going outside with wet hair will cause a cold or that the north wind brings colds and flu. Most of us have been told that sitting in a draft is the best way to catch a cold. None of these theories has been proven. Colds and flu are caused by viruses, and more than 150 of them have been identified. Although there is no cure, the symptoms can be treated fairly successfully. If you have poor nutrition, you are fatigued, or your emotions are disturbed, you may be more susceptible to these viruses when you are exposed to them, or the resulting illness may be more severe. The reason we get colds and flu predominantly during the winter months is due partially to the stress of winter, but more to the fact that we are indoors, with closer contact with other people who can spread the viruses. The time lag between being exposed to the virus and getting the symptoms is rather short—one to four days usually. But remember that a cold is contagious one or two days prior to showing symptoms, so you can be pass it on without even knowing you have it (or someone else has it and is giving it to you). The onset of a cold is usually gradual, with symptoms increasing over 2–4 days, while the onset of the flu is often very fast, becoming full blown within 6–12 hours after the initial symptoms.

Cold symptoms. Colds frequently start off with symptoms of a sore throat, vague fatigue, muscle aches, and a feverish feeling without an elevated body temperature. More common symptoms appear as you develop congestion. Bacterial infections may complicate a cold, with ear, sinus, or throat infections being most common. A runny nose, coughing, sneezing, nasal/sinus congestion, laryngitis, and a sore throat usually round out the symptoms. For most people a cold lasts 5–7 days.

Flu symptoms. Flu is very much like a cold, but the symptoms are usually more generally distributed than the localized respiratory symptoms of a cold. Often the first symptom is a fever. The runny nose, cough, and sore throat are generally less prominent or common than with a cold, but the symptoms of headache, fever, and body aches are increased. The duration of the flu is usually 5–14 days.

Sneezing. Sneezing is a protective reflex that is important in clearing foreign objects from the airways. Why it sometimes occurs or persists in association with respiratory infections is not clear. With allergies, it is a very common symptom. Treatment options are limited, and no drugs are truly specific for this problem. In allergic disease sneezing can often be attributed to the presence of histamine, and the antihistamine class of drugs is effective (see page 66) to relieve this symptom. For sneezing associated with colds or flu, it is not clear whether or not the antihistamines offer any real help.

Sore Throat

Sore throats result from several different causes but are most commonly caused by an infection. Numerous organisms, including primarily bacteria and viruses, may be the cause. There are no over-the-counter antibiotics to treat bacterial throat infections, and nothing is effective against viruses, the most common cause of sore throat; so only symptomatic relief can be applied. If the pain is severe or persistent (or a high fever is present), a bacterial (strep) infection is likely, and you must see a doctor to obtain effective antibiotic treatment. The products listed below reduce the discomfort and provide minor, temporary relief. Even candy lozenges or cough drops are effective for many people in soothing a sore throat. Gargles can be used and do supply some relief, but by far the best treatment is to take ibuprofen (or aspirin or acetaminophen, see Chapter 2, pages 21–24) and use an anesthetic lozenge for topical soothing/anesthetic effects.

Key Active Ingredients for Sore Throat

Dyclonine. Dyclonine is a local anesthetic with a rapid onset of effect and good absorption through the skin or mucous membranes. It is safe, due to low side effects, including only the very rare development of allergic reactions. It is particularly well suited for topical oral use. **Pregnant women, nursing mothers, and seniors:** no special problems or needs for its topical use.

Benzocaine. Introduced 85 years ago, benzocaine was one of the first, and is still one of the best, local anesthetics. It is used in many diverse formulations for surface pain relief, and also for relief of itching. It is very poorly absorbed through the skin and mucous membranes, making it quite safe for use. Few adverse effects are associated with its use, though occasionally a person may become allergic. **Pregnant women, nursing mothers, and seniors:** no special problems or needs for its topical use.

Sore Throat (Topical Pain Relief, Lozenges)

FIRST CHOICE *for seniors, adults, children*

Generic name: Dyclonine HCl

Adult Dose: 3 mg

Pediatric dose: 1.2 mg

Brand names: Children's Sucrets, Sucrets Maximum Strength Sore Throat Lozenges

Reasons: Dyclonine is an effective topical anesthetic, which is especially good for sore throat. It has very low toxicity and can be used repeatedly (by lozenge) for temporary relief of sore throat.

Cautions: None of significant concern.

Sore Throat (Topical Pain Relief)

SECOND CHOICE *for seniors, adults, children*

Generic name: Benzocaine

Dose: 5–32 mg

Brand names: Cepacol Troches, Chloraseptic Cool Mint, Soretts, Spec-T, Thorets, Vicks Throat Lozenges

Reasons: As described above, benzocaine is the best overall general local anesthetic useful for treating various types of local pain. Though dyclonine is the first choice for sore throat, benzocaine is also very effective and useful for this indication.

Cautions: There is a slightly increased potential for toxic side effects or for developing allergies to benzocaine compared with dyclonine, but it is still a good choice for relief of sore throat pain.

Cough

A common symptom for both colds and flu, a cough can be caused by various other problems as well—asthma being one of the more common initiators. If coughing produces mucous or phlegm it is best not to suppress it, as it is serving the purpose of clearing out the airways. If the cough is just irritating and results in nothing being coughed up, it can be suppressed using one of several over-the-counter agents available. In some states, codeine, which is a cough suppressant (low doses) and analgesic (in larger doses) can be purchased over the counter, but in many states it is restricted to prescription-only availability. Since codeine is no more effective than dextromethorphan (the first choice for cough), and has the potential to become addicting, it will not be recommended; but it is effective and can be used in place of dextromethorphan. If a cough does not clear up spontaneously within a few days, the cause of the problem must be determined and treated. The most common cause is post-nasal drip as a result of sinus infections. Decongestants or antibiotics are needed to correct this problem. A second cause of more chronic coughs is asthma, which again requires appropriate treatment to correct the situation. Acid reflux is the third most common cause of cough. Acid from the stomach gets into the lower esophagus and induces cough. In this case, the use of antacids or surgical correction will cure the cough.

Safe, Effective Ingredients for Cough

Dextromethorphan. Dextromethorphan is a cough suppressant introduced in 1958 and widely used. It is the best in this class and seems to be equivalent in effectiveness even to the prescription-only agents. It acts on the cough control center in the brain to relieve persistent dry cough. It has little sedative effect, but some individuals may experience drowsiness. It should not be used to suppress a cough that produces phlegm, because it may prolong a chest infection by preventing the clearance of sputum by the cough mechanism. **Pregnant women:** safety not established, but no evidence of risk. **Nursing mothers:** passes into the breast milk. **Seniors:** reduce dose or increased side effects likely. **Drug interactions:** alcohol or sedatives—increased risk of sedation; MAOI (monoamine oxidase inhibitor) drugs (certain antidepressants)—increased excitation, possible fever.

Diphenhydramine. Diphenhydramine is a commonly used antihistamine, which has additional properties, including some cough suppressive activity. It is available in a number of products, but is not the best agent for this use. If you cannot tolerate dexromethorphan for some reason, you could substitute diphenhydramine for cough suppression. **Pregnant women:** safety not established, but no evidence of risk. **Nursing mothers:** passes into the breast milk. **Seniors:** reduce dose or increased side effects likely. **Drug interactions:** alcohol, sedatives—increased sedation; anticholinergics—increased effects; MAOI (monoamine oxidase inhibitor) drugs (certain antidepressants)—risk of acute hypertension (high blood pressure).

Codeine. Codeine has the potential to be habit forming, and most states have regulated this ingredient so it is available only by prescription. It is very effective (at least equal to dextromethorphan) and is generally safe in the amounts used to suppress cough. It should not be used for a prolonged period, due to possible side effects (constipation) and the potential for addiction. **Pregnant women:** safety not established, but no evidence of risk. **Nursing mothers:** passes into the breast milk. **Seniors:** reduce dose or increased side effects possible. **Drug interactions:** alcohol, sedatives—increased sedation; MAOI (monoamine oxidase inhibitor) drugs (certain antidepressants)—risk of acute hypertension (high blood pressure).

Expectorant Ingredients

Guiafenisen. Guiafenisen is the only effective over-the-counter drug available in this class. Expectorants are used to help liquify and dilute phlegm and mucous so that they can be coughed up and cleared from the airways. None of these agents is dramatically effective, and in fact, drinking plenty of liquids is just as effective (or maybe even more so) than taking the drug. Its use is recommended because many of the cough suppressants have it anyway, and it is so safe that arguments against its use are not convincing. **Pregnant women, nursing mothers, and seniors:** there is no evidence suggesting special needs or any problems.

Cough Suppressants Plus Expectorant
(Oral Cough Syrups, Liquids, and Tablets)

FIRST CHOICE *for all ages*

Generic name: Dextromethorphan *and* guiafenisen

Dose: Dextromethorphan, 30 mg; guiafenisen, 50–400 mg

Brand names: Cremacoat 1, Delsym, DM Cough, Genatuss DM, Halotussin-DM, Mediquell (Chewy Squares), Mytussin DM, Naldecon Senior DX, Nycoff, Pertussin ES, Queltuss, Robitussin DM, Sorbutuss, St. Joseph Cough Suppressant for Children, Sucrets 4-Hour Cough Suppressant, Vicks Children's Cough

Reasons: Simple cough can be suppressed very effectively without the extra ingredients contained in many cough products. In those listed, the best active ingredient that is safe and effective is used, and in nearly all, the only ingredient recognized to help liquify mucous (expectorant) is also used. In many cases, the dose of the cough suppressant and/or the expectorant is less than optimal, but at least the ingredients are appropriate.

Cautions: Because a cough can be a symptom of many other illnesses that require treatment, you should only treat it for a few days. If it does not resolve itself or becomes worse, consult your doctor. The drugs in these preparations are safe, and only a low incidence of minor side effects is associated with their use.

Nasal/Sinus Congestion (Oral Agents)

Three agents in this class are recognized as effective and safe for over-the-counter use. The best of the three is *pseudoephedrine hydrochloride (HCl)*, found in many preparations. If this agent does not work well for you, or causes unpleasant side effects, the next agent of choice is *phenylpropanolamine hydrochloride*. This causes a higher incidence of excitation as a side effect, and it is the only ingredient recognized safe and effective for use as an appetite suppressant, so this effect makes it less desirable. Finally, *phenylephrine hydrochloride* is an effective alternative found in many decongestant preparations.

Preferred Decongestant Ingredients

Pseudoephedrine HCl. Widely used, pseudoephedrine reduces nasal and sinus congestion by shrinking swollen blood vessels. This makes it prone to cause nervous system stimulation, including nervousness, anxiety, tremor, disturbed sleep, and restlessness. However, of all agents in this class, it is the least likely to cause these effects. **Pregnant women:** safety not established, some risk probable. **Nursing mothers:** passes into the breast milk. **Seniors:** reduce dose or increased side effects likely. **Drug interactions:** antihypertensives—decreased effects; MAOI (monoamine oxidase inhibitor) drugs (certain antidepressants)—risk of acute hypertension (high blood pressure).

Phenylpropanolamine HCl. Phenylpropanolamine is another widely used decongestant that shrinks blood vessels. It is more likely to produce additional undesirable effects, including increased heart rate, raised blood pressure (the first symptom of which is usually a severe headache), palpitations, and sleep disruption. Although side effects are minimal when used properly, since this drug is found in many combination cold products (and in diet aids), overdoses are fairly frequent due to lack of awareness of its widespread occurrence in multiple products that may be used simultaneously. An additional side effect, appetite suppression, makes this drug the only over-the-counter diet aid available. Together, these uses make this drug the fifth most frequently used over-the-counter remedy in the country. However, it probably should not be taken by people with hypertension (high blood pressure) except by topical application to the nose. **Pregnant women:** safety not established, some risk probable. **Nursing mothers:** passes into the breast milk. **Seniors:** reduce dose or increased side effects likely. **Drug interactions:** antihypertensives—decreased effects; MAOI (monoamine oxidase inhibitor) drugs (certain antidepressants)—risk of acute hypertension (high blood pressure).

Phenylephrine HCl. Phenylephrine is a common decongestant for nasal/sinus symptoms of congestion. It is also commonly used by the topical (direct) route of application. It has more potential for side effects on heart rate and blood pressure (increases both) and on the nervous system (anxiety, tremor, insomnia) than the other two decongestant agents. **Pregnant women:** some risk likely, animal studies show teratogenic (fetal malformation) effects, but no evidence in humans to suggest this occurs. **Nursing mothers:** passes into the breast milk. **Seniors:** reduce dose or increased side effects likely. **Drug interactions:** antihypertensives—decreased effects; MAOI (monoamine oxidose inhibitor) drugs (certain antidepressants)—risk of acute hypertension (high blood pressure)

Nasal/Sinus Congestion Alone
(Oral Use for Decongestion)

FIRST CHOICE *for seniors, adults, children*

Generic name: Pseudoephedrine

Dose: 30–60 mg

Maximum: 120 mg (long acting)

Brand names: Cenafed, Congestac, Dorcol Children's Decongestant, Drixoral Non-Drowsy Formula, Fedahist Expectorant (and Pediatric), Genaphed, Oranyl, Robitussin PE, Sudafed (and Children's liquid), Sudanyl

Reasons: If possible, single ingredient medications should be used if the symptoms are limited to congestion. In this case, antihistamines are frequently combined with decongestants for treatment of colds and flu. This results in unnecessary drowsiness and drying of the mouth and nose, causing more discomfort for treatment of an illness where these agents probably are not effective anyway. For allergies, the antihistamine ingredient contributes significantly to the relief of symptoms, but for viral infections they seem to add only to the side effects (which, however, at times is useful to make the patient sleepy and rest easier).

Cautions: Pseudoephedrine has the greatest margin of safety of all the drugs in this class and is also very effective. It can have side effects, including raised blood pressure, increased heart rate, and occasional nervousness.

Nasal/Sinus Congestion Alone
(Oral Use for Decongestion)

SECOND CHOICE *for seniors, adults, children*

Generic name: Phenylpropanolamine *or* phenylephrine

Dose: Phenylpropanolamine, 12.5–37.5 mg; phenylephrine, 5–10 mg

Brand names: Codimal Expectorant, Conex, Myminic Expectorant, Naldecon EX Pediatric, Poly-Histine Expectorant, Propagest, Triaminic Expectorant, Triphenyl Expectorant

Reasons: Both phenylpropanolamine and phenylephrine are effective decongestants and are used in a variety of products. They are frequently combined with other drugs to give multisymptom relief and to try to balance their side effects against those of the other drugs in the combination, especially antihistamines.

Cautions: Both of these drugs have a somewhat increased incidence of side effects compared to pseudoephedrine, with hypertension (increased blood pressure) being most prominent. Nervous system and kidney side effects are also rarely seen. The most common side effect is headache, which if caused by an increase in blood pressure, can be severe.

Sinus Headache (Oral Use, Combination Drug)

FIRST CHOICE *for seniors, adults, children*

Generic name: Ibuprofen (analgesic) *and* pseudoephedrine (decongestant)

Dose: Ibuprofen, 200–400 mg; pseudoephedrine, 30–60 mg

Brand names: Advil Cold & Sinus, Co-Advil, Motrin IB Sinus

Reasons: A combination of the best analgesic (for pain) and the best decongestant make this product the most effective and convenient way to handle sinus headaches (congestion with headache).

Cautions: No special problems; just the normal incidence of potential side effects based on the individual ingredients.

Sinus Headache (Oral Use, Combination Drug)

SECOND CHOICE *for seniors, adults, children*

Generic name: Acetaminophen *or* aspirin (analgesic) *and* pseudoephedrine *or* phenylpropanolamine (decongestant)

Dose: Acetaminophen, 325–650 mg; aspirin, 325–650 mg; pseudoephedrine, 30–60 mg; phenylpropanolamine, 12–37 mg

Brand names: Allerest No Drowsiness, Bayer Children's Cold, Bayer Select Sinus Pain, Bayer Select Head Cold, Drinophen, Dristan Maximum Strength, Emagrin Forte, Excedrin Sinus, Fiogesic, Naldegesic, Oranyl Plus, Ornex, Sinarest No Drowsiness, Sine-Aid Maximum, Sine-Off Maximum Strength No Drowsiness, Sinutab Maximum Strength without Drowsiness, St. Joseph Cold Tablets for Children, Sudafed Sinus, Super Anahist, Tylenol Sinus Maximum Strength

Reasons: All of these products combine the second or third choice analgesic agents with the first or second choice decongestant, making them good choices but somewhat inferior to the first choice in both safety and effectiveness. They are combinations of widely used and safe ingredients; so they are a good alternative if convenience or cost considerations make the first choice less attractive.

Cautions: There are no special problems or effects that need to be noted here. The side effects are those that would be expected from the individual agents used.

Nasal Congestion—Topical Therapy

Best Ingredients for Topical Decongestants

Oxymetazoline. A particularly good decongestant for topical use, oxymetazoline acts by constricting (shrinking) the blood vessels in the nose. It has a longer-lasting effect than most others, so dosing only twice a day is effective. Side effects are milder and less common than with many other decongestants (oral and topical). It may be irritating if used frequently or for too long. Topical agents are generally safe for use in all populations. **Pregnant women, nursing mothers, and seniors:** no evidence of special considerations. **Drug interactions:** antihypertensives—decreased effects; MAOI (monoamine oxidase inhibitor) drugs (certain antidepressants)—risk of acute hypertension (high blood pressure).

Xylometazoline. Xylometazoline is a locally acting nasal decongestant which shrinks blood vessels in the nose. It has a shorter duration of effect than oxymetazoline and a higher incidence of side effects, including headache, palpitations, and drowsiness. Topical agents are generally safe for use in all populations. **Pregnant women, nursing mothers, and seniors:** No evidence of special considerations. **Drug interactions:** antihypertensives—decreased effects; MAOI (monoamine oxidase inhibitor) drugs (certain antidepressants)—risk of acute hypertension (high blood pressure).

Phenylephrine. Phenylephrine is a common decongestant for nasal/sinus symptoms of congestion. It is also used orally. It has a greater potential for side effects on heart rate and blood pressure (increases both) and on the nervous system (anxiety, tremor, insomnia) than the other two drugs listed. Topical agents are generally safe for use in all populations. **Pregnant women, nursing mothers, and seniors:** no evidence of special considerations. **Drug interactions:** antihypertensives—decreased effects; MAOI (monoamine oxidase inhibitor) drugs (certain antidepressants)—risk of acute hypertension (high blood pressure).

Nasal Congestion Alone (Topical Relief of Congestion)

FIRST CHOICE *for seniors, adults, children*

Generic name: Oxymetazoline

Adult dose: 0.05% conc.

Pediatric dose: 0.025% conc.

Spray or mist: Afrin 12-Hour, Allerest, Chlorphed-LA, Coricidin, Dristan Long-Lasting, Duramist Plus, Duration, 4-Way Long Lasting, Neo-Synephrine Maximum 12 Hour, Nostrilla Long Acting 12 Hour, NTZ Long Lasting, Sinarest, Sinex-LA

Solution or drops: Afrin 12-Hour, Genasal, NTZ Long Lasting, Twice-A-Day

Pediatric (drops): Afrin 12 hr Pediatric

Reasons: Oxymetazoline is an effective, fast-acting, long-lasting nasal decongestant when applied topically to the nose. Best overall in this class, it also seems to be less likely to produce rebound congestion (an effect sometimes seen after prolonged use, or when discontinuing the use of these decongestants, when stopping the medication actually causes the congestion to reoccur).

Cautions: None of special concern.

Nasal Congestion Alone (Topical Relief of Congestion)

SECOND CHOICE *for seniors, adults, children*

Generic name: Xylometazoline *or* phenylephrine

Adult dose: xylometazoline, 0.05–0.1% conc.; phenylephrine, 0.2–0.5% conc.

Pediatric dose: phenylephrine 0.125% conc.

Nasal sprays/mists: Alconefrin 25, Doktors, Dristan (spray), Dristan Menthol, 4-Way Fast Acting (regular and menthol),

Myci-Spray, Neo-Synephrine (Regular and Extra), Nostril 1/2% Regular, Otrivin, Rhinall, Sinex, Xylometazoline Hydrochloride

Nasal drops/solutions: Alconefrin (25 and 50), Doktors, Neo-Synephrine (Regular and Extra), Otrivin, Rhinall-10

Pediatric drops: Neo-Synephrine Pediatric, Otrivin Pediatric

Reasons: Both of these drugs are good alternatives for the first choice agent. They are effective, and wide use has demonstrated their safety.

Cautions: None of major concern—an advantage of topical therapy.

Cough and Congestion Together

Because cough and congestion frequently occur together, it is common to combine the active ingredients into one medication. Congestion and sinus drainage into the throat often irritate the throat and cause a cough. Combination products with these two drugs (and sometimes an expectorant, described earlier) are available in a wide variety of forms (and, as described below, also in combination with analgesics and antihistamines).

Effective Ingredients for Combination Drugs

See the individual ingredient descriptions of cough suppressants and decongestant agents on pages 54 and 57.

Guiafenisen. Although some authorities are not convinced of the usefulness of this expectorant, it has been shown to be effective (when used in adequate doses) to help loosen mucous and help the airways. An adequate intake of liquids is also very important, and in many cases will accomplish the desired end alone. However, since the drug is very safe and may help to liquify and loosen mucous, it is recommended for use in conjunction with cough suppressants and decongestants (which may cause thickening of the mucous) to get the maximum possible benefit.

Cough/ Congestion Combination Agents
(Oral Use, Liquids and Tablets)

FIRST CHOICE *for seniors, adults, children*

Generic name: Dextromethorphan (cough suppressant) *and* pseudoephedrine (decongestant) *and* guiafenisen (expectorant)

Dose: Dextromethorphan, 5–30 mg; pseudoephedrine, 20–60 mg (120 mg long lasting); guiafenisen, 100–400 mg

Brand names: Ambenyl-D Decongestant Cough Formula, Conar Expectorant, Cough Formula with Expectorant, Dorcol Children's, Formula 44D Decongestant Cough Mixture, Noratuss II Expectorant, Novahistine DMX, Ru Tuss Expectorant, Sudafed Cough

Reasons: Dextromethorphan is a very effective cough suppressant without other significant effects, making it an excellent choice. The optimal dose of 30–60 mg works for several hours. Pseudoephedrine is the first choice of decongestants, so this combination has the two best drugs to accomplish the relief of symptoms. The expectorant is extra insurance, to help liquify and loosen mucous and clear the airways.

Cautions: The combination of dextromethorphan, pseudoephedrine, and guiafenisen is relatively selective in its effect and only rarely causes problems. Overall, low toxicity and superior effect make this drug combination a good choice.

Cough/Congestion Combination Drugs
(Oral Use, Some with Expectorant)

SECOND CHOICE *for seniors, adults, children*

Generic name: Dextromethorphan (cough suppressant) *and* phenylpropanolamine (decongestant) *and* guiafenisen (expectorant)

Dose: Dextromethorphan, 15–30 mg; phenylpropanolamine, 12–37 mg; guiafenisen, 50–400 mg

antihistamines a...
ment of allergies
Each of several ...
teristics that may
for another. There
mended here as be
common cold, and
Administration) ha...
some benefit. This
new data with othe...
was found on cold s...
has had some ques...
caused an increase i...
lamine. It is almost su...
recommended anywa...
of the popular combi...
(including Contac Ni...
Night). If a preparatio...
cold or flu (it may pr...
runny nose or itching ...
combinations are given ...

Headache, Congesti...

C...

THIRD CHOI...

Generic name: Ch...
acetaminophen (analgesic/...
phenylpropanolamine (d...
(cough suppressant)

Dose: Chlorpheniram...
mg; pseudoephedrine, 30–60...
mg); dextromethorphan, 15–3...

Brand names: Bayer S...
Contac Severe Cold Formula,...
Cold & Cough Medicine, Ty-...
Viro-Med

Brand names: With expectorant: Naldecon DX (Adult, Children's, Pediatric), Primatuss Cough Mixture 4D, Robitussin CF, Tussex Cough

Without expectorant: Bayer Cough Syrup for Children, Conar, Snaplets-DM (granules), Triaminic DM, Tricodene Pediatric

Reasons: These products combine the second choice decongestant with the first choice cough suppressant. They are effective and safe when used as directed. Some contain the expectorant, guiafenisen, to help liquify and loosen secretions that might build up in the airways.

Cautions: People with high blood pressure probably should not take these medications. The decongestant, phenylpropanolamine, can increase blood pressure, especially if more than the recommended dose is used. Since this drug is found in many products, this extra dose may be taken without realizing it.

Flu and Colds—Combination Drugs

This category is full of products that take the shotgun approach to treatment. Since it is always best not to take more drugs than are necessary, only the combinations with the top ingredients for each symptom are recommended.

**Headache, Congestion, Cough, Fever
(No Drowsiness Formula)**

FIRST CHOICE *for seniors, adults*

Generic name: Ibuprofen (for pain/fever) *and* pseudoephedrine *and* dextromethorphan (for cough)

Dose: Ibuprofen, 200–400 mg; pseudoephedrine, 30–60 mg; dextromethorphan, 15–30 mg

Brand names: None. Take ibuprofen along with the appropriate decongestant or decongestant/cough formulation (see pages 66 and 70).

Reasons
ducts for this i
maximum effec

Cautions.
in its effects an
superior effectiv

Headache, Cong

SE

Generic name
ephedrine (for cong
some with expectora

Dose: Acetar
30–60 mg; dextromet

Brand names:
Cough Formula, Co
Tylenol Cold No Drow

Reasons: These
with the best cough su
the analgesic is not the
phen is the choice of a
susceptible to stomach
mended for children.

Cautions: This co
effects and only rarely ca
effectiveness make this co

A Note About Antihist

Antihistamines are not rec
to provide significant bene
However, many of the mo
antihistamine as a main in

Reasons: These products contain the first choice ingredient for all of the categories except the analgesic (ibuprofen is recommended over acetaminophen) or in some, the decongestant (pseudoephedrine is recommended over phenylpropanolamine). They are therefore very effective and a good choice overall if all of the symptoms are present and relief is desired by the shotgun approach. They provide the maximum possible profile of relief.

Cautions: As with all such combinations, realize that multiple drugs mean the potential for multiple side effects. In particular, in the combination agents that contain an antihistamine, users must be aware of the possibility of drowsiness or attention-deficit problems and should not operate any machinery or vehicles.

Allergies

More than 26 million people in the United States (about one in ten people) recognize their allergic disease, and even more people suffer, but don't even realize that they have allergies. At times it is difficult to separate allergies from cold and flu symptoms. In general, the following symptoms are typical for those persons suffering from an allergic reaction:

- Dark, swollen bags under the eyes
- Irritated, red, itchy, watery eyes
- Sneezing
- Runny nose with thin, clear watery discharge
- Itching of the roof of the mouth

Fever, chills, and muscle aches are only rarely seen with allergy. The most common allergy is "hayfever," which is not due to hay and has no fever. It results from allergic responses to molds that grow in hay and many other places and causes the variety of symptoms noted above. Contrast with these, the symptoms of colds and flu, which are generally: sneezing—it is rare with the flu but not uncommon for a cold—fever, chills, and muscle aches; and a runny nose, with thick, yellow or green discharge.

Antihistamines are the drugs of choice for allergic reactions. There are a large number of these drugs and it is difficult to tell them apart. They have broad effects, and side effects are common, but rarely serious. Stimulants (caffeine) can be used to help counter the drowsiness or sedation most of them cause. Taking them with food can reduce the stomach or intestinal side effects that some people experience. They are also used as an ingredient in many cold and flu medications, but the evidence that they provide any benefit for flu or colds is weak. They are basically all equally effective if the proper dose is given, but individuals do find that one or another may work better for them. The recommendations given reflect the results of studies of preference by the majority, more on the basis of lower side effects and a superior duration of effect than differences in effectiveness (which are small, if any).

Safe and Effective Antihistamines

Chlorpheniramine. In use for over 30 years, chlorpheniramine is best overall in this class. It reduces sneezing, runny nose, and itching (eyes and skin), and can reduce swelling and redness. It works by blocking the effects of chemicals produced by the body in response to allergic reactions. Overall, this drug has lower drowsiness and other side effects characteristic of this class of drugs (except for some new "nonsedating" prescription-only antihistamines). **Pregnant women:** not usually recommended because of lack of data. **Nursing mothers:** no evidence of risk to infant. **Seniors:** reduced dose may be desirable or increased side effects may occur. **Drug interactions:** alcohol, sedatives—increased sedation; anticholinergics—greater effects; MAOI (monoamine oxidase inhibitor) drugs (certain antidepressants)—risk of hypertension (high blood pressure).

Brompheniramine (dexbrompheniramine). These drugs are so similar to chlorpheniramine that they are indistinguishable from it. They have the same effects and profile.

Diphenhydramine. Diphenhydramine is one of the oldest and most common antihistamines. Due to widespread and long-time use, it is recognized as very safe. It was the first highly successful drug to be switched from prescription-only to over-the-counter availability. It exhibits a high incidence of characteristic side effects; so much so that it is also used as a sleep-inducing aid, a cough suppressant, and antinausea drug. **Pregnant women:** no evidence of risk. **Nursing mothers:** no evidence of risk to infant, but passes into breast milk. **Seniors:** reduced dose may be desirable or increased side effects may occur. **Drug interactions:** alcohol, sedatives—increased sedation; anticholinergics—increased effects; MAOI (monoamine oxidase inhibitor) drugs (certain anti-depressants)—risk of hypertension (high blood pressure).

Triprolidine. Triprolidine is another of the potent, very effective members of the antihistamine class. It is of a different chemical group than the others, but it is indistinguishable in effectiveness and side effects (although somewhat more sedating, like diphenhydramine). It is recommended for those who do not obtain satisfactory relief with the others or experience unacceptable side effects from the other agents in this class. Only by trying it can you determine if it will be better for you. **Pregnant women:** no data. **Nursing mothers:** no data. **Seniors:** reduced dose may be desirable or increased side effects may occur. **Drug interactions:** alcohol, sedatives—increased sedation; anticholinergics—increased effects.

Antihistamines Not Recommended

There are quite a number of other antihistamines available. If the agents recommended here do not give satisfactory relief, you could try one of the others. Each class has different characteristics that may make it better for one individual than for another. The recommendations are based on results of comparison studies, and only the best are included. Only one, *doxylamine,* has some question raised about safety, since large doses caused certain types of cancer in rats to increase. It is almost surely not cancer-causing in humans, but for this reason, it is not recommended. It is an ingredient in many of the popular combination agents for cough, colds, and flu (including Nyquil, Contac Nighttime, Nycold, Pertussin, and Quiet Night.

=====

Allergy Symptoms—Hives/Skin Rash, Sneezing, Watery Eyes (Oral Use)

FIRST CHOICE *for seniors, adults, children*

Generic name: Chlorpheniramine *or* brompheniramine

Dose: Chlorpheniramine, 2–4 mg (8–12 mg, long acting); brompheniramine, 2–12 mg

Tablets: Aller-Chlor, Chlor-Trimeton (long acting and maximum strength), Dimetane, Pfeiffer's Allergy, Teldrin

Liquids: Aller-Chlor, Chlor-Trimeton, Dimetane

Reasons: For relief of respiratory allergic symptoms or for hives or allergic skin reactions, the best treatment is chlorpheniramine alone. A single-ingredient agent is preferred. All over-the-counter antihistamines have sedation or drowsiness as a potential side effect. The least sedating of these is chlorpheniramine. It also has a good duration of effect, so it doesn't have to be taken in as large a dose or as often in order to be effective.

Cautions: As with all antihistamines, there is a possibility of sedation, and adjustments must be made should this side effect occur. Otherwise, this agent is safe and effective.

Allergy Symptoms—Hives/Skin Rash, Sneezing, Watery Eyes (Oral Use)

SECOND CHOICE *for seniors, adults, children*

Generic name: Diphenhydramine *or* triprolidine

Dose: Diphenhydramine, 25–50 mg; triprolidine, 1.25–2.5 mg

Tablets: Actidil, Aller-Max, Banophen, Benadryl 25

Liquids: Actidil, Genahist, Nidryl, Phendry

Reasons: These second choice products are also plain antihistamines. They have ingredients that are somewhat more sedating than the first choice listed above, but diphenhydramine has a very long history of use by millions of people and is considered to be safe and effective.

Cautions: These agents have a significant potential to induce drowsiness and/or decrease alertness. The cautions against operating machinery or performing tasks requiring a high level of alertness must be followed.

Allergy Symptoms—Congestion, Sneezing, Watery Eyes, Itchy Throat (Oral Use)

FIRST CHOICE *for seniors, adults, children*

Generic name: Chlorpheniramine *or* dexbrompheniramine (antihistamine) *and* pseudoephedrine (decongestant)

Dose: Chlorpheniramine *or* dexbrompheniramine, 2–4 mg; pseudoephedrine, 30–60 mg

Brand names: Chlor-Trimeton Decongestant, Co-Pyronil 2, Dallergy-D, Dexophed, Dorcol Children's Formula, Drixoral, Fedahist, Isoclor, Myfedrine Plus, Napril, Pedia Care Cold, Ryna, Sinutab Allergy Formula, Sudafed Plus

Reasons: These products combine the best antihistamine with the best decongestant to provide safe and effective symptom relief.

Cautions: Observe the usual precautions with these classes of drugs. The antihistamines must always be considered as potentially sedating. The decongestant may cause side effects relating to stimulation of the nervous system or rare increases in blood pressure. Follow label directions.

Allergy Symptoms—Congestion, Sneezing, Watery Eyes, Itchy Throat (Oral Use)

SECOND CHOICE *for seniors, adults, children*

Generic name: Triprolidine *or* diphenhydramine (antihistamine) *and* pseudoephedrine (decongestant)

Dose: Triprolidine, 2.5 mg (*or* diphenhydramine, 25–50 mg); pseudoephedrine, 30–60 mg

Brand names: Actagen, Actifed, Allerfrin OTC, Aprodine, Benadryl Decongestant, Benylin D, Coryban D, Genac, Triofed

Reasons: These products are the second choice in this class because although the decongestant (pseudoephedrine) is the best choice, the antihistamine ingredient is the second choice. Triprolidine and diphenhydramine are somewhat more sedating and less preferred overall than the first choice agents described above. Many people will find these drugs completely acceptable, since not everyone experiences the drowsiness that antihistamines tend to cause.

Cautions: As with all such products containing antihistamines, the main side effect to watch for is the drowsiness. Do not drive or operate machinery if drowsiness occurs. In some cases, caffeine may help overcome mild drowsiness, but caution must be exercised, and the label instructions followed carefully.

Allergy Symptoms with Headache (Oral Use)

FIRST CHOICE *for seniors, adults, children*

Generic name: Ibuprofen (analgesic) *and* chlorpheniramine (antihistamine) *and* pseudoephedrine (decongestant)

Dose: Ibuprofen, 200–400 mg; chlorpheniramine, 2–4 mg; pseudoephedrine, 30–60 mg

Brand names: None. Take ibuprofen with the first choice allergy agents noted above. No combination agents have ibuprofen.

Reasons: Although ibuprofen is somewhat more expensive than aspirin or acetaminophen, it is the most effective analgesic and is safer to use than aspirin. It relieves pain, reduces fever, and counters inflammation. Take it with meals to reduce stomach upset (if necessary).

Cautions: Ibuprofen may cause stomach upset (nausea or vomiting) and rarely can cause ulcers (much less than aspirin). Diarrhea or constipation may also occur rarely. Patients with kidney disease should consult a physician before using these products. Ibuprofen may interact with antihypertensive (blood pressure) drugs, diuretics (water pills), alcohol, antacids, and anticoagulants. Consult your physician if you take these medications. **Pregnant women:** not usually recommended, due to lack of experience.

Nursing mothers: no evidence of risk to infant. **Seniors:** reduced dose may be desirable.

Allergy Symptoms with Headache (Oral Use)

SECOND CHOICE *for seniors, adults, children*

Generic name: Acetaminophen (analgesic) *and* chlorpheniramine *or* dexbrompheniramine (antihistamine) *and* pseudoephedrine *or* phenylpropanolamine (decongestant)

Dose: Acetaminophen, 325–650 mg; chlorpheniramine *or* dexbrompheniramine, 2–4 mg; pseudoephedrine, 30–60 mg (*or* phenylpropanolamine, 12–40 mg)

Brand names: Bayer Select Allergy Sinus, Codimal, Comtrex (Allergy-Sinus), Drixoral Plus, Kolephrin, PhenAPAP Sinus Headache & Congestion, Sine-Off Maximum Strength Allergy/Sinus, Singlet, Sinulin, Sinutab Maximum Strength, TheraFlu Flu and Cold Medicine, Tylenol Allergy Sinus

Reasons: These products combine the best antihistamine with the best, or second best, decongestant. The analgesic is the second choice (acetaminophen instead of ibuprofen), but it is effective for the intended purpose. These drugs are very effective combination agents and most likely will provide maximum relief.

Cautions: Since these are combination agents, there is the possibility of multiple side effects and side effects from interactions among the different drugs. Most important is the side effect of drowsiness, which is common with all drugs containing antihistamines.

Allergy Symptoms with Headache (Oral Use)

THIRD CHOICE *for seniors, adults, children*

Generic name: A combination from each of the following agents:

Analgesic: Ibuprofen *or* acetaminophen *or* aspirin

Antihistamine: Chlorpheniramine, brompheniramine, dex-brompheniramine, diphenhydramine, *or* triprolidine

Decongestant: Pseudoephedrine, phenylpropanolamine, *or* phenylephrine

Brand names: Virtually any. The distinctions begin to blur when you get down this far and one or more of the components is the second or third choice for its category.

Asthma

For many years, asthma was mistakenly thought to be due to neurosis or hypochondria (induced by the mind). On the contrary, it is a serious condition where the airways and lungs become inflamed, preventing the efficient exchange of air (oxygen in, carbon dioxide out). The death rate due to asthma has increased steadily for several years and is the most common cause of hospitalization for children. Asthma is also the leading cause of missed days from work and school. There is no cure, but excellent treatment is available. The cause cannot always be determined, but in many cases asthma is an allergic reaction that occurs in the lungs. Widely recognized symptoms of asthma include wheezing, cough, and shortness of breath, which may be triggered by cold air, smoke, exertion, stress, pollution, and various allergens.

Asthmatics cannot usually tell how sick they are until they get into serious trouble. The symptoms of wheezing and shortness of breath do not occur until lung function is seriously compromised and the patient is in danger. For this reason, there are now inexpensive hand-held devices (peak flow meters) that allow the objective monitoring of lung function. These devices can show a decrease in lung function long before the individual notices the problem. The goal is to prevent serious attacks of asthma by treating the inflamed, swollen, blocked airways early. Again, prevention is more effective than treatment to reverse the attack. This is best accomplished by working out a good regimen with a doctor. For rare attacks, some over-the-counter drugs are available for use as noted below.

Active Ingredients for Asthma

Epinephrine. Epinephrine is a hormone produced by the body in response to stress which makes you "ready to go" (to run or fight). It is used as a drug for several purposes, including opening the breathing tubes (airways) in asthma. It is topically effective and acts very quickly. Because it also constricts blood vessels, it can be used as a decongestant. It is not as selective as newer prescription-only drugs for use as a bronchodilator, so it produces more side effects, including nervousness and palpitations. **Pregnant women:** may cause problems. **Nursing mothers:** passes into breast milk. **Seniors:** reduced dose may be desirable or increased side effects may occur. **Drug interactions:** cardiac (heart) drugs—various interactions (talk with physician); antidiabetic drugs—decreased effects.

Ephedrine. Ephedrine is a drug that acts by stimulating the release of a natural hormone to shrink blood vessels and relax muscles in the airways, resulting in decongestion and opening of the airway (bronchodilation). Newer and more effective drugs are available only by prescription. **Pregnant women:** safety not established. **Nursing mothers:** passes into breast milk. **Seniors:** reduced dose may be desirable, or even better yet, just avoid this drug if possible. **Drug interactions:** cardiac (heart) drugs (especially digitalis)—various interactions (talk with physician); antihypertension drugs (blood pressure) decreased effects; MAOI (monoamine oxidase inhibitor) drugs (certain antidepressants)—risk of acute hypertension.

Theophylline. For treatment of asthma, theophylline relaxes the muscles in the airways and stimulates breathing and heart rate. It has additional beneficial effects for the treatment of asthma, but to obtain the maximum benefit, blood levels of this drug must be carefully adjusted. Since effective and toxic doses vary among individuals, but are always close together, the dose must be controlled to avoid toxic effects. A wide variety of adverse effects, including nausea, headache, indigestion, and nervousness occur when too much is given. **Pregnant women:** safety not established. **Nursing mothers:** passes into breast milk. **Seniors:** reduced dose may be desirable or increased side effects may occur. **Drug interactions:** many drugs alter the blood level of theophylline with concurrent use. Do not use without a doctor's care if you have heart disease or diabetes.

Asthma Symptoms—Cough or Wheezing (Aerosol Use)

FIRST CHOICE *for seniors, adults, children*

Generic name: Epinephrine

Dose: 0.16 mg / spray

Brand names: AsthmaHaler, Breatheasy, Bronitin Mist, Bronkaid Mist, Medihaler-Epi, Primatene Mist

Reasons: There is only one active ingredient for this indication contained in all of the available products. The choice can be based on cost or on the preferred dosage for maximum personal convenience.

Cautions: Asthma can be a life-threatening disease and requires diagnosis and treatment by a doctor if it is serious. This medication is for temporary, occasional use only.

Asthma Symptoms—Cough or Wheezing (Oral Use, Tablets or Capsules)

FIRST CHOICE *for seniors, adults, children*

Generic name: Ephedrine *and* theophylline

Dose: Ephedrine, 24 mg; theophylline, 100 -130 mg

Brand names: Amesec, Bronkaid, Primatene, Primatene-NS

Reasons: The only active ingredients recognized as safe and effective are contained in all of the oral asthma preparations. In some states a number of other preparations (not listed) also contain phenobarbital in combination with ephedrine and theophylline. This ingredient is a depressant and is not recommended. If your state does not permit its sale over the counter, many other brands are available without the phenobarbital. They are just as good as those listed (check the ingredients).

Cautions: As with all self-treatment of potentially serious diseases, in particular the oral treatment of asthma, great care must be taken to use the medication correctly. The ingredients used in these preparations (especially theophylline) can be very toxic when taken to excess and are only effective when given properly. Physicians using this drug monitor the blood level to be sure the dosage is correct for the individual.

5

Gastrointestinal System

The gastrointestinal (G.I.) system includes organs and structures involved in the intake and processing of food and excretion of solid wastes. A number of symptoms and diseases can affect the G.I. system, and a group of effective, safe, and useful over-the-counter drugs are available to treat these problems. This chapter reviews, describes, and recommends the best agents for treatment of nausea and vomiting, hangover, heartburn and indigestion, diarrhea, constipation, hemorrhoids, and a few other related ailments.

Few symptoms cause as much discomfort or cause us to modify our activities as much as those affecting our stomach and bowels. These organs and the regulation of the habits related to their functions, including eating, are central to the enjoyment of life. Treatment of symptoms or modification of G.I. functions can be very difficult because the large number of products in this group leads to confusion over choosing appropriate drugs. Recommended agents are discussed first based on their common symptoms, route of administration, and speed of effect. Then, individual problems and their treatment are covered.

Antacids and Specific Indications for Their Use

There are a bewildering number of antacids to choose from. They are all the same in the ultimate action, but they differ in their ability to neutralize stomach acid and thereby reduce the pain of ulcers, heartburn, and indigestion. The side effects vary for the different agents, some tending to cause diarrhea and others constipation. For this reason, the best antacids are generally a combination of two agents, one that tends to induce diarrhea and one that tends to cause constipation, so that the opposing effects counter each other and the drugs have no noticeable side effects. Antacids should be taken about one hour after a meal for maximum benefit. When taken on an empty stomach, the antacid effect lasts about 20 minutes, whereas if taken after a meal, the effect may last 2–3 hours. Liquid, gel, or suspension preparations are preferred because the medicine is already in the best form (liquid) to counter stomach acid. Tablets are less effective and, if used, they must be chewed thoroughly in order to be of maximum benefit. Some antacids act very fast, but their effects are very short, and they must be taken often. Continuous or prolonged use of antacids can cause problems with nutrient levels (vitamins and minerals), so they should be used only as needed.

ULCERS. The exact cause of ulcers has not been determined. What is clear is that the normally protective surface of the stomach, esophagus, or small intestine is eroded or damaged, allowing stomach acid to irritate the underlying tissue and cause a severe burning-type pain. Some of the most recent medical research suggests that a local bacterial infection may be the root of the problem, and curing this infection cures the ulcer. Until the cause or a cure can be established, the treatment of ulcers remains symptomatic, using either antacids to neutralize the acid, or drugs that reduce the production of stomach acid. Only the antacids are currently available without a prescription. In most studies on patients with ulcers, the vigorous, continuous use of antacids has been shown to be as effective as the drugs that block the production of acid. This is true for both relieving the pain and in the rate of healing.

HEARTBURN/INDIGESTION. About 10% of people suffer from heartburn daily, and another 33% occasionally. This burning sensation in the chest, sometimes followed by a bitter taste in the mouth, is not connected to the heart, but is a stomach acid problem. The valve that separates the stomach from the esophagus (the pipe that food goes through from the mouth to get to the stomach) does not work well and allows stomach acid to get into the esophagus. This problem is relieved by antacids, which act by neutralizing the acid. As noted below, a number of antacids are effective and useful for this problem.

In addition to taking antacids as needed, there are several other steps that can ease the problem of frequent heartburn: eat smaller amounts of food at one time (to reduce free acid content in the stomach); lose weight (to take pressure off the valve that lets the acid leak into the esophagus); eat at least 3–4 hours before lying down or going to bed (so the stomach is empty and doesn't put pressure on the valve); stop smoking (it irritates the esophagus); raise the head of your bed 3–4 inches (to help the valve keep the acid from backing up); and avoid certain foods that tend to make the problem worse—fatty, spicy, acidic foods, red wine, and coffee (that stimulate more acid or irritate the tissue). Finally, calcium stimulates acid secretion, so antacids containing calcium may aggravate the problem and should be avoided.

Antacids—Major Players

Magnesium hydroxide. This popular, effective (potent), fast-acting antacid and laxative is rarely found as a single ingredient. It works best when used in combination with aluminum hydroxide. It is excellent for single, occasional use alone. **Pregnant women:** no evidence of risk. **Nursing mothers:** no evidence of risk to infant. **Seniors:** no special problems. **Drug interactions:** alcohol—increased stomach irritation, decreased benefit; also interferes with the absorption of numerous drugs.

Aluminum hydroxide. This is not as good an antacid since it tends to induce constipation. However, aluminum hydroxide and magnesium hydroxide counter each others' effects, making this combination the best overall antacid available. Possible phosphate deficiency can occur with prolonged use. **Pregnant women:** safety not established. **Nursing mothers:** no evidence of risk to infant. **Seniors:** reduce dose or increased constipation likely. **Drug interactions:** interferes with absorption of numerous drugs, including anticoagulants, digitalis, tetracycline, penicillamine, and steroids.

Calcium carbonate. This is a potent antacid, but the calcium is absorbed and may cause kidney problems if used too frequently or in large doses. It also has a constipating effect and therefore is not recommended for routine use. Calcium also stimulates acid secretion, so this antacid may aggravate the problem at the same time it is helping. **Pregnant women, nursing mothers, and seniors:** no evidence of data for special needs.

Brand names include Alamag, Marblen, Titrilac Plus, and Tums Extra in liquid form. Tablets are sold under Alka-Mints, Alkets, Amitone, Calcilac, Chooz, Diatrol, Dicarbosil, Di-Gel, Dimacid, Equilet, Genalac, Glycate, Mallamint, Marblen, Noralac, Rolaids Calcium Rich, Titracid, Titralac, Tums, and Tums-E-X.

Sodium bicarbonate. This effective, fast-acting antacid should not be used in large or repeated doses because it is absorbed (taken into the blood) and can be toxic. Sodium bicarbonate also contains a lot of salt, which is not good, especially for people with hypertension. It can be used occasionally as a single-use agent for rapid, short antacid effects (baking soda or as Alka-Seltzer and other brands). **Pregnant women, nursing mothers, and seniors:** no special needs or cautions. People with high blood pressure should avoid the extra salt.

Indigestion, Heartburn, and Ulcers (Liquid) High-Potency or Concentrated Formulas

FIRST CHOICE *for seniors, adults, children*

Generic name: Aluminum hydroxide *and* magnesium hydroxide

Dose: Aluminum hydroxide, 80–120 mg conc./ml; magnesium hydroxide, 60–90 mg/ml.

Brand names: Almacone II, Anta Gel-II, Gelusil II, Maalox Plus Extra Strength, Maalox TC, Mylanta II, Simaal 2 Gel

Reasons: These products contain the best antacids in concentrated form. A lower strength antacid can be used if these high-potency effects are not needed, but it may be better to just reduce the dose of these high-potency products. (See the second choice for the "regular" potency versions of these same products.)

Cautions: None of special concern; may rarely cause diarrhea or constipation in selected persons, but generally well tolerated and free of problems.

Indigestion, Heartburn, and Ulcers (Liquid) Regular Strength Formulas

SECOND CHOICE *for seniors, adults, children*

Generic name: Aluminum hydroxide *and* magnesium hydroxide

Dose: Aluminum hydroxide, 30-60 mg/ml conc.; magnesium hydroxide, 20-40 mg/ml.

Brand names: Almacone, Alma-Mag, Aludrox, Anta Gel, Camalox, Di-Gel, Gelusil, Kolantyl, Maalox, Magna Gel, Magnesia and Alumina, Mi-Acid, Mintox, Mintox Plus, Mygel, Mylanta, Rulox, Simaal Gel, WinGel

Reasons: These products provide a lower dose of the preferred antacid combination for relief of heartburn. They combine the most effective agents and are generally free of either constipating or diarrhea-inducing side effects.

Cautions: There are few side effects or problems; may interact with other drugs to prevent their complete absorption.

Indigestion, Heartburn, and Ulcers High-Potency or Regular Potency Formulas (Chewable)

THIRD CHOICE *for seniors, adults, children*

Generic name: Aluminum hydroxide *and* magnesium hydroxide

High-potency dose: Aluminum hydroxide, 400–600 mg; magnesium hydroxide, 300–400 mg

Regular dose: Aluminum hydroxide, 160–260 mg; magnesium hydroxide, 75–200 mg

Brand names: (High-Potency) Gelusil II, Maalox Extra Strength, Maalox TC, Mylanta II, Rulox #1; (Regular) Almacone, Alma-Mag #4, Camalox, Creamalin, Gelusil, Maalox, Magnatril, Mylanta, Rulox #1, WinGel

Reasons: Tablets are a less efficient form of antacids, but can be very effective if used correctly. These products contain the best ingredients in this class and have the lowest overall potential for side effects.

Cautions: Safe and effective when chewed well to break the tablet into small pieces. To avoid overdose, which may induce either diarrhea or constipation in some people, follow label directions.

Indigestion, Heartburn, and Ulcers (Fast Acting Liquids with Brief Effect)

FOURTH CHOICE *for all ages*

Generic name: Sodium bicarbonate

Dose: See label

Liquids: Alka Seltzer Effervescent Antacid, Citrocarbonate

Tablets: Bell/ANS, Gaviscon, Soda Mint, Sodium Bicarbonate, Triconsil

Reasons: Fast acting and effective, sodium bicarbonate is a useful antacid for occasional quick relief.

Cautions: Sodium bicarbonate should not be used repeatedly or frequently because the ingredients are absorbed and can cause adverse effects by shifting the balance of ions in the blood and by adding too much salt to the body. People on salt-restricted diets or those with hypertension (high blood pressure) should avoid this antacid.

Antiemetics and Specific Indications for Their Use

Antiemetics prevent or reduce nausea and vomiting. Compared with full-blown nausea, the unpleasantness of hunger, fatigue, and thirst pale to insignificance. There are three products to choose from in this category for the prevention and treatment of nausea, motion sickness (car, boat, airplane), and vomiting. Each is an antihistamine, which means they have additional effects, including causing drowsiness in some people. The choices recommended are based on the ability of each agent to provide relief to the largest number of people, the best being effective in about 85% of people.

MOTION SICKNESS, NAUSEA, AND VOMITING. Nausea and vomiting can be caused by a number of problems, including infections, reactions to food, medications, and alcohol, as well as a host of more serious intestinal conditions. It is also common during early pregnancy. Optimal treatment includes avoiding solid foods and drinking clear liquids. For morning sickness (pregnancy) none of the agents has been proven safe, but the least amount of risk is associated with the use of dimenhydrinate (third choice overall) because the active ingredient has been used by millions of people over many years without problems.

Active Ingredients for Nausea and Vomiting

Meclizine. Meclizine is an antihistamine, but is only used for its antiemetic effects. It prevents and treats motion sickness, nausea, and vomiting. It does have more side effects than the usual antihistamines (used for allergies), including drowsiness, dry mouth and—rarely—blurred vision. A slower onset of effect and longer duration of activity means it should be taken in advance of travel for maximum effect. **Pregnant women:** may cause problems—it is a teratogen (causes fetal malformations) in animals, but no evidence in humans to suggest this occurs. **Nursing mothers:** pas- ses into breast milk. **Seniors:** no special problems, but reduced dose may be better to prevent side effects. **Drug interactions:** alcohol and sedatives—increased sedation.

Cyclizine. Cyclizine is an antihistamine of the same chemical class as meclizine, exhibiting many of the same properties. Used as an antiemetic, it is very effective. Its side effects are similar to meclizine, but perhaps slightly greater in frequency. The reduced alertness caused by this drug was reversed by caffeine in human laboratory testing, so this option can be considered if drowsiness is a problem. **Pregnant women:** may cause problems—it is a teratogen in animals (causes malformations of the fetus), but no evidence in humans to suggest problems. **Nursing mothers:** no data. **Seniors:** no special problems, but reduced dose may be better to prevent side effects. **Drug interactions:** alcohol and sedatives—increased sedation.

Dimenhydrinate. Another antihistamine used for antiemetic effects, this is another form of the well-known antihistamine, diphenhydramine. Long experience and wide use show it is very safe, but somewhat less effective than the other antiemetics. It works well for many people. **Pregnant women:** no evidence of risk in humans. **Nursing mothers:** passes into breast milk. **Seniors:** No special problems, but reduced dose may be better to prevent side effects. **Drug interactions:** alcohol and sedatives—increased sedation.

Motion Sickness, Nausea, and Vomiting

FIRST CHOICE *for seniors, adults, children*

Generic name: Meclizine

Dose: 25–50 mg

Brand names: Bonine, Dizmiss, Meclizine

Reasons: In large-scale testing (thousands of service men crossing the ocean by ship during World War II) as well as in laboratory testing, this ingredient was most effective.

Cautions: As with all such medications, drowsiness is possible and the precautions on the label should be followed. Animal studies suggest fetal malformations may occur, but no evidence of their occurrence in humans has been found. To be safe, meclizine should not be used by pregnant women.

Motion Sickness, Nausea, and Vomiting

SECOND CHOICE *for seniors, adults, children*

Generic name: Cyclizine

Dose: 50 mg

Brand names: Marezine

Reasons: In large-scale testing (thousands of service men crossing the ocean by ship during World War II) and laboratory testing, this ingredient was second in effectiveness.

Cautions: As with all such medications, drowsiness is possible and the precautions on the label should be followed. In animal tests cyclizine induced some birth defects, so it should not be used by pregnant women.

Motion Sickness, Nausea, and Vomiting

THIRD CHOICE *for seniors, adults, children*

(FIRST CHOICE for morning sickness if medication cannot be avoided)

Generic name: Dimenhydrinate

Dose: 50 mg

Brand names: Calm-X, Dramamine, Marmine, Tega-Vert, Triptone

Reasons: This agent induces more drowsiness than the other two and is somewhat less effective. Some of the other side effects (dry mouth, and so on) seem to be lower with this drug than the other antiemetics, so you have some choice on this count. Because it has been used for many years by millions of people, this agent is believed to have the lowest risk of adverse effects on the fetus.

Cautions: As with all such medications, drowsiness is possible, and especially with this agent. Follow the precautions on the label.

Antiflatulents

Flatulence is a common problem with unpleasant though no serious symptoms. Gases, often smelling like rotten eggs and/or highly flammable, are formed in the intestines and produce pressure (cramping) and a "bloated" feeling. Particularly after eating certain foods and during times of illness this problem may be quite common, although some people have the problem fairly consistently without specific inducers. Medical treatment (antibiotics) may be helpful for persistent problems, but occasional flatulence will resolve itself, or can be treated symptomatically as needed with the over-the-counter anti-gas aides recommended below.

Active Ingredient for Gas

Simethicone. Use of this over-the-counter drug is somewhat controversial. Authorities disagree on the extent to which it is effective in combatting gas. Simethicone is used for its antifoaming and water-repellent properties and for pretreatment of patients for X-ray procedures, where it has been shown effective in reducing gas in the intestine. It probably does reduce the symptoms of excess gas and provides some relief. It is also very safe.

Generic name: Simethicone

Dose: 80–125 mg

Maximum: 500 mg/day

Brand names: Brite-Life Gas Relief, Gas-X, Gas-X Extra Strength, Maalox Anit-gas, Mylanta Gas

Reasons: These products contain the only effective agent for anti-gas effects that is safe and effective, and in a dose that is large enough to have the desired effect.

Cautions: None of any concern.

Diarrhea

Acute, simple diarrhea usually lasts for a few days and is most often caused by a bacterial or viral infection, food poisoning, anxiety, or a reaction to food(s), medication, or alcohol. Treatment for diarrhea includes avoiding milk and dairy products (because many people find them hard to digest and irritation of the bowel is increased) and drinking plenty of clear liquids (to prevent dehydration and the complications arising from this common problem). There are several good products available over the counter to treat this problem. They do not address the cause—since it is usually unknown and often cannot be treated specifically anyway—but symptomatic treatment until the problem corrects itself is very satisfactory. The best medication is a new over-the-counter product (previously prescription only), *loperamide*. It is just as effective as the prescription product Lomotil, and is safer and does not have the habit-forming potential of Lomotil.

There is no evidence that the duration of an infectious diarrheal illness is increased by treating the symptoms. Other products do not act as quickly nor are they as effective in as many people as loperamide, including the old stand-by, Pepto-Bismol. For traveler's diarrhea (a frequent problem on trips, especially to foreign countries), there is good evidence that prophylactic (preventive) treatment with Pepto-Bismol will reduce the incidence of diarrhea. This is because in addition to antidiarrheal activity, the active ingredient in Pepto-Bismol (*bismuth subsalicylate*) has some antibacterial effects; and bacterial infections are often the cause of traveler's diarrhea (different, new organisms in the food and water of the country or area being visited).

Antidiarrheal Active Ingredients

Loperamide. A relatively new drug (about 15 years of use) recently switched to over-the-counter availability from prescription only. It reduces loss of water and salts caused by diarrhea and slows bowel activity. It is fast acting and is usually effective after only one dose. Adverse effects are rare because the drug is not absorbed, but acts locally. Cramps or constipation may occur (rarely) as side effects. It is the best agent in this class. Studies show its use does not prolong the disease process. **Pregnant women:** safety not established. **Nursing mothers:** slight amount passes into the breast milk. **Seniors:** no special problems. **Drug interactions:** none known.

Attapulgite. This is another effective and safe agent for treatment of diarrhea, which is well tolerated. It has a slower onset of effect than loperamide, and several doses and some patience may be required before the anti-diarrheal effects are seen. Since it acts by direct local effects on the water content of the bowel, there are virtually no side effects. **Pregnant women, nursing mothers, and seniors:** no problems or considerations for special populations. **Drug interactions:** none known.

Bismuth subsalicylate. This antidiarrheal agent is quite effective for traveler's diarrhea, because in addition to reducing the number and frequency of stools, it has some antibacterial effects (a frequent cause of traveler's diarrhea). It can be used prophylactically (in anticipation that diarrhea may occur) to prevent diarrhea. It is not as effective as loperamide once diarrhea has started. Side effects are few (some constipation), but other unpleasant features of this agent include the possible blackening of the tongue and stool and it may also cause ringing in the ears for some users. It is a close relative of aspirin, so when combined with that drug, the side effects, including ringing in the ears, become much more common. **Pregnant women:** no data, but since it is an aspirin-like ingredient, best to avoid if possible. **Nursing mothers:** passes into milk. **Seniors:** no special problems. **Drug interactions:** may interfere with absorption of numerous drugs; aspirin adds to its side effects and toxicity due to similar effects.

Diarrhea (Liquid and Tablet)

FIRST CHOICE *for seniors, adults, children*

Generic name: Loperamide

Dose: 2–4 mg

Brand names: Brite-Life Anti-diarrheal, Imodium A-D (caplet and liquid), Loperamide, Maalox Anti-diarrheal

Reasons: Loperamide is the best antidiarrheal agent available, and in fact appears to be as good as any of the prescription agents for this indication. Unlike the prescription agents, it is not habit forming. It is generally very effective following a single dose.

Cautions: Rare side effects, probably not distinguishable from the diarrhea it is used to treat.

Diarrhea (Liquid and Tablet)

SECOND CHOICE *for seniors, adults, children*

Generic name: Attapulgite or bismuth subsalicylate

Dose: Attapulgite, 300–750 mg; bismuth subsalicylate, 13–16 mg/ml

Liquids: Diar-Aid, Diasorb, Infantol Pink, Kaopectate, Pepto-Bismol, Percy Medicine

Tablets: Diasorb, Kaopectate, Pepto-Bismol, Rheaban

Reasons: Not as effective as loperamide, these products are useful but may require several doses before taking effect. Bismuth subsalicylate is also useful as a preventive therapy for traveler's diarrhea, due to some antibacterial action (a common cause of traveler's diarrhea).

Cautions: There are few to no side effects expected with the use of attapulgite. The bismuth subsalicylate is a relative of aspirin and when taken with aspirin, or in large or repeated doses, may induce overdose side effects typical of aspirin, including ringing in the ears, fever, and nausea or vomiting.

Hemorrhoids

A common affliction, especially after age 40, over 50% of the people in the United States have some form of hemorrhoids. The majority of these people do not have symptoms and get along well without any treatment. Hemorrhoids are inflamed, enlarged blood vessels in the anorectal area, which may cause pain, burning, itching, and general discomfort. The objective of treatment is to reduce the discomfort and allow healing. Both internal and external hemorrhoids are common and can cause symptoms, but they may also occur without inducing symptoms. In addition to the symptomatic treatment described here, an improvement in bowel habits, particularly keeping the area clean and dry, will reduce the problem. Bed rest and sitz baths (sitting in a pan of warm water, often with salts added) are frequently the most beneficial treatments overall.

The exact cause of hemorrhoids is unknown, but they are increased by pregnancy, long periods of standing or sitting, coughing, sneezing, vomiting, and exertion. To protect the area and reduce discomfort, *white petrolatum* (petroleum jelly) and *zinc oxide* are both excellent. For temporary relief of flare-ups, the following section describes the most effective and safe agents available over the counter. Stool softeners may also be very helpful (see page 108) to reduce straining for a bowel movement and to soften the stool. Suppositories and ointments are commonly used for local relief of symptoms. Both work well, with the suppositories appearing to be a little better early in the course of treatment, but both requiring about two or three weeks for good control. In this class of drugs, there is considerable disagreement and lack of firm scientific data to support many of the products currently on the market. One such ingredient is the "live yeast cell derivative" contained in Preparation H and Wyanoids. Recent clinical testing of this yeast derivative failed to show effectiveness, and more tests are needed if the companies want to continue to use this ingredient in their products.

Effective Ingredients for Hemorrhoids

Benzocaine, pramoxine, diperodon, tetracaine. These are all local anesthetics used in various products for hemorrhoids. It is very difficult to make any product judgments about these, since no good comparison studies are available. All are probably effective, and differences in duration or efficacy are not likely to be very great. More study is needed for this indication and this class of drugs. **Pregnant women:** safety not established, but due to topical nature of use, risk if any is minimal. **Nursing mothers:** no data. **Seniors:** no special problems.

Zinc oxide, petrolatum, cocoa butter. These are the main ingredients used in hemorrhoid preparations to protect and soothe the inflamed area. Applied after cleaning the area, they are the best of the agents for protecting and allowing healing while reducing irritation. They are very safe for use. **Pregnant women, nursing mothers, and seniors:** special needs are not a consideration.

Hemorrhoids (Topical Treatment for Pain Plus Protectant)

FIRST CHOICE *for seniors, adults, children*

Generic name: Benzocaine, dibucaine, pramoxine, diperodon, *or* tetracaine *and* zinc oxide, petrolatum, *or* cocoa butter

Dose: See label

Ointments: Anusol, Hemet Rectal, Hemocaine, Hemorid, Medicone Rectal, Nupercainal, Pontocaine, Primaderm-B, Rectagene Medicated

Suppositories: Anocaine Hemorrhoidal, Hemet Hemorrhoidal, Hem-Prep, Medicone Rectal

Reasons: These products contain safe, effective ingredients to deal with the most common symptoms of hemorrhoids. Local anesthetic helps relieve pain and itching through effects on the pain endings (nerves) that register the pain, and protectants serve to keep irritating substances from the tender, inflamed area. Very little distinction can be made among these agents, but some have additional ingredients, such as aloe, which may or may not provide extra benefit (the data are not convincing).

Cautions: These products are applied locally and therefore have very little potential to produce toxic effects. Local irritation or redness may occur occasionally, but this is hard to distinguish from the symptoms of the disease being treated. The local anesthetics as a group have the potential to induce allergic reactions, or if used heavily and absorbed, some general effects (restlessness, tremor, drowsiness), but these are very rare.

Hemorrhoids (Topical Treatment for Pain Relief Only)

SECOND CHOICE *for seniors, adults, children*

Generic name: Benzocaine *or* pramoxine

Dose: See label

Brand names: Americaine (ointment), Fleet Relief Anesthetic Hemorrhoidal (ointment), Lanacane (cream), Non-steroid Protofoam (foam), Tronolane (cream and suppository)

Reasons: These products are specialized, providing symptom relief only by the action of local anesthetics that block the pain signals. The first choice agents also provide some protection and soothing effects, which is why they are recommended first. For simple relief of pain and itching, these products are acceptable alternatives.

Cautions: The local anesthetics have the potential to induce allergic reactions, but this is rare. If burning, redness, itching, or swelling occur, discontinue use. Topical application rarely produces any other side effects.

Hemorrhoids (Topical Treatment with Protectant Only)

THIRD CHOICE *for seniors, adults, children*

Generic name: Zinc oxide, cocoa butter, *or* petrolatum

Dose: See label

Ointments: Vaseline Pure Petroleum Jelly

Suppositories: Anusol, Calmol 4, Nupercainal

Reasons: These agents all provide the protection that helps allow healing and reduces irritation of the inflamed tissue from the passage of stools. In many cases, a conscientious effort to keep the area clean and apply protectants will allow the inflammation to subside on its own.

Cautions: None expected; these products are very safe.

Constipation

A change in bowel habits that results in the infrequent passage of hard stools can be attributed to a number of possible causes, including inadequate fiber in the diet, insufficient water intake, drugs, travel, or stress and a change in diet. Many agents are available to treat this symptom, and the main criterion for selection is how fast you want the drug to work. Different classes of laxatives may act within a few hours or not for a few days. The most effective and safe laxatives are divided into groups by the amount of time needed to provide relief. The most desirable laxative is the slowest acting, because it has the least side effects or potential for producing problems. Several related products all have the same property: they increase the bulk and soften the consistency of the stool by absorbing and retaining water in the intestine. For a faster effect, the intermediate acting (several hours to overnight) stimulant agents can be used. These agents should not be used repeatedly because they can become habit forming as the intestine becomes less active on its own and depends on the stimulation provided by the medication to perform its function. For relief of constipation within an hour or two, topically applied agents as well as certain oral agents can effect a very rapid (watery) evacuation of the intestine. The rapid but somewhat unpredictable timing of these agents and the frequent side effects (especially cramps) make them generally unpleasant to use.

In addition to the use of drugs, the following measures will help get you on a regular schedule and relieve the problem: increase your intake of water, step up physical activity, develop a regular routine for both eating and voiding, increase your fiber intake, and avoid constipating foods (like rice, chocolate, and bananas).

Active Ingredients in Laxatives

Methylcellulose. This has been a commonly used laxative for more than 40 years. It is not absorbed, but acts locally in the intestine to absorb water (up to 25 times its own volume) to soften and increase stool volume. This product should be taken with adequate amounts of water or other liquids. Methylcellulose can also be used to treat diarrhea, where it acts to firm stools, again by regulating the water content of the stool. It has a rather slow onset of effect, but is the preferred agent for constipation if fast action is not required. It is also used in diet aids, to add bulk to the stomach, and in the eye for artificial tears to relieve dryness. **Pregnant women:** no evidence of risk, assumed safe. **Nursing mothers:** no reason to expect problems. **Seniors:** no special problems. **Drug interactions:** may reduce absorption of numerous other drugs.

Bran or psyllium. These bulk-forming laxatives are derived from the milling of wheat or from plant seeds, respectively. Each has been used for more than 50 years. Taken as a powder or as granules dissolved in water, they soften the stool and increase stool bulk by absorbing water. They can also be used for diarrhea, by regulating the water content of the stool (they absorb about 25 times their volume of water). Rarely, they may dry up and cause plugging of the bowel if the person's liquid intake is insufficient. Bloating and excess gas may occur in some cases. **Pregnant women:** no evidence of risk, assumed safe. **Nursing mothers:** no reason to expect problems. **Seniors:** no special problems. **Drug interactions:** may reduce absorption of numerous other drugs.

Polycarbophil. This agent acts as a sponge to bind water, and as such it can serve as treatment for either diarrhea or constipation. It acts by readjusting the water content to a "normal" consistency. It is not absorbed, so it has very little toxicity except what can be attributed to local effects (possible bloating or pain). It has a very slow onset of effect; often up to 48 hours is required before it is effective. One major disadvantage is that a large dose is required for the desired effect. **Pregnant women:** no evidence of risk, assumed safe. **Nursing mothers:** no reason to expect problems. **Seniors:** no special problems. **Drug interactions:** may reduce absorption of numerous other drugs.

Docusate. This product has minimal laxative effects, but is included here because it is widely used as a stool softener. It is very useful to maintain a moist stool and to help prevent straining to have a bowel movement. This effect is important for hemorrhoid sufferers and for anyone who has frequent problems with constipation. It is generally not effective until one to three days after starting therapy. It interacts with some of the laxatives (especially the stimulant types). **Pregnant women:** no evidence of risk, assumed safe. **Nursing mothers:** no reason to expect problems. **Seniors:** no special problems.

Mineral oil. This is a thick oil and lubricant that is not very well absorbed, and therefore helps to soften the feces and pass the stool through the intestine. It interferes with the absorption of fat and nutrients, so should not be used over a prolonged period of time. It is safe and effective for occasional use. **Pregnant women:** no evidence of risk, assumed safe. **Nursing mothers:** no reason to expect problems. **Seniors:** no special problems. **Drug interactions:** may reduce absorption of numerous other drugs, vitamins, and minerals.

Phenolphthalein. This is one of the widely used and common "stimulant" laxatives. The stimulant laxatives are usually effective in 6–8 hours. It is generally taken at bedtime, and the bowel movement occurs on awakening. Depending on the dose, side effects include cramping and diarrhea. This drug acts on the mucosa of the intestine and since it is absorbed into the blood, may have a longer duration of effect than the locally acting agents. **Pregnant women:** safety not established. **Nursing mothers:** no data. **Seniors:** no special problems, but reduced dose may be better.

Bisacodyl. Bisacodyl is a powerful stimulant laxative, related to phenolphthalein, which normally acts in 6–12 hours. It helps to keep the stool soft and stimulates muscle contraction to move the stool through the bowel. It can also cause stomach irritation. Regular or long-term use can upset normal bowel function, leading to diarrhea and loss of needed nutrients, especially potassium. Bisacodyl can also be given rectally for a faster effect (15–60 minutes). **Pregnant women:** safety not established. **Nursing mothers:** no data. **Seniors:** reduce dose or increased side effects likely. **Drug interactions:** with antacids and milk—increased stomach irritation noted.

Senna. Senna is similar in use and effects to phenolphthalein and bisacodyl, with its major effects on the large intestine. Another of the stimulant class of laxatives, it takes effect in 6–8 hours. Like the other agents that are absorbed, if taken in too high a dose senna may cause side effects, including diarrhea and loss of nutrients. **Pregnant women:** safety not established. **Nursing mothers:** no data. **Seniors:** reduce dose or increased side effects likely.

Casanthrol or cascara sagrada. Obtained from tree bark, these drugs have long been used as cathartic agents. They are similar to senna and the other stimulant laxatives in use and effects. They usually cause a single soft or semifluid evacuation of the bowel about 8 hours after dosing. **Pregnant women:** safety not established. **Nursing mothers:** passes into breast milk. **Seniors:** reduce dose or increased side effects likely.

Magnesium sulfate (or citrate). These salts of the mineral, magnesium, have a very rapid onset of effect, usually within 1–3 hours. At lower doses, the onset may be somewhat slower. They cause a dramatic retention of water in the intestine and increase the speed of transit through the bowel, resulting in a watery evacuation of the bowel. They are not absorbed, so like most other fast-acting agents, they have low side effects. If sufficient liquids are not ingested, there can be local effects including diarrhea, cramps, and dehydration. **Pregnant women:** no evidence of risk. **Nursing mothers:** no evidence of risk. **Seniors:** no special problems.

Castor oil. This is another of the heavy oils that acts directly on the small intestine to stimulate a prompt and thorough evacuation of the bowel. It also reduces nutrient absorption, so it should not be used repeatedly. Side effects are typical of this group (diarrhea, bloating, and so on) due to local effects that stimulate bowel activity. **Pregnant women:** no evidence of risk. **Nursing mothers:** no evidence of risk. **Seniors:** no special problems.

Glycerin. Glycerin is another agent that acts through its physical property of being able to absorb water to relieve constipation. It can be somewhat dehydrating if fluid intake is not sufficient. It also can act as an irritant to stimulate the bowel, especially if given by suppository. **Pregnant women:** no evidence of risk. **Nursing mothers:** no evidence of risk. **Seniors:** no special problems.

Constipation (Laxatives for Oral Use)
Slow Acting, Effective in 1–2 Days

FIRST CHOICE *for seniors, adults, children*

Generic name: Methylcellulose, psyllium, *or* polycarbophil

Dose: See label

Tablets: Disoplex, Equalactin, Fiberall, FiberCon, Mitrolan (chewable), Naturacil (chewable)

Liquids and powders: Cillium, Citrucel, Cologel, Effersyllium, Fiberall (natural), Hydrocil Instant, Konsyl, Konsyl-D, L.A. Formula, Metamucil (instant and flavored), Modane Bulk, Natural Vegetable, Perdiem Fiber, Reguloid (flavored and natural), Serutan, Siblin, Syllact, Syllamalt, V-Lax

Reasons: Slow in onset, but very safe and effective, these are the preferred products for treatment of constipation. They act locally by retaining or adjusting the water content in the bowel to soften the stool and prevent straining while voiding.

Cautions: These agents are safe and effective when used as directed. Always in the case of constipation, you must drink large amounts of water or other liquids to maintain good hydration and allow the agents to do their job by adjusting the water content of the stool.

Constipation (Laxative and Softener) Oral Use
Intermediate Acting, Effective in 6–8 Hours

FIRST CHOICE *for seniors, adults, children*

Generic name: Docusate *or* mineral oil (softener) *and* phenolphthalein (laxative)

Dose: Softener, 60–230 mg; laxative, 60–200 mg

Tablets/capsules: Colax, Correctol, Disolan, Doxidan, Ex-Lax extra gentle, Feen-A-Mint, Femilax, Laxcaps, Modane Plus, Phillip's LaxCaps, Unilax

Liquids: Agoral, Kondremul with Phenolphthalein

Reasons: These are the products of first choice in the stimulant or intermediate action group. They are generally effective in 6–8 hours. They have direct stimulatory effects on the intestine to move stool through more quickly, while it is still moist. A softening agent is included with most of these drugs to prolong the softening effect.

Cautions: Since these agents all act by direct stimulation of the intestine, there is a danger that the bowel may become "lazy" and not function well on its own. For this reason, repeated use of these agents will eventually cause problems. They are for occasional, fast-acting relief. Side effects include cramps; pain; the potential for diarrhea and loss of fluids, electrolytes, or other nutrients, particularly if the dose is too large.

Constipation (Laxative and Softener for Oral Use)
Intermediate Acting, Effective in 6–8 Hours

SECOND CHOICE *for seniors, adults, children*

Generic name: Senna *or* casanthrol (laxative) *and* docusate (softener)

Dose: Laxative, 187 mg (senna); 30 mg (casanthrol); softener, 50-100 mg

Tablets/capsules: Afko-Lube Lax, Constiban, Dialose Plus, Diocto-K-Plus, Dioctolose Plus, Di-Sosul Forte, Diothron, Disanthrol, Docusate with Casanthranol, DSMC Plus, D-S-S Plus, Genasoft Plus, Gentlax S, Peri-Colace, Peri-Dos, Pro-Sof Plus, Regulace, Senokot-S

Liquids/syrups: Diocto C, Diocto-K-Plus, Docusate with Casanthranol, Peri-Colace

Reasons: These products also contain safe and effective stimulant ingredients and a stool softener. They differ little from the first choice agents.

Cautions: Since these agents all act by direct stimulation of the intestine, there is a danger that the bowel may become "lazy" and not function well on its own. For this reason, repeated use of these agents will cause problems. They are for occasional, fast-acting relief. Possible side effects include cramps, pain, and the potential for diarrhea (causing the loss of fluids, electrolytes or other nutrients), particularly if the dose is too large.

**Constipation (Laxative Alone for Oral Use)
Intermediate Acting, Effective in 6–8 Hours**

THIRD CHOICE *for seniors, adults, children*

Generic name: Phenolphthalein

Dose: 60–130 mg

Brand names: (Tablets—some chewable) Alophen, Espotabs, Evac-U-Gen, Evac-U-Lax, Ex-Lax, Lax-Pills, Modane, Modane Mild, Phenolax, Prulet

Reasons: These products are recommended as the third choice agents in this class primarily because they lack a softening agent. They contain a very effective stimulant laxative, which acts overnight, but the first choice agents also have an ingredient to help soften the stool. This gives a longer lasting benefit and prevents the problem from recurring the next day or so. Phenolphthalein is fine if the problem is acute and if one bowel movement is all that is necessary to return to regularity. If the problem requires a longer term adjustment in habits, the softener can provide additional transition time to get back to a normal schedule.

Cautions: Use all stimulant-type laxatives according to instructions. Repeated use can lead to a lazy bowel that relies on the drug to function, and may actually cause the constipation to become worse. They are for relief of acute problems only. If the problem persists more than a week, other solutions must be sought. All stimulant laxatives have the potential to induce cramps or abdominal pain and even diarrhea if the dose is too large.

Constipation (Laxative Alone for Oral Use)
Fast Acting, Effective in 1–3 Hours

FIRST CHOICE *for seniors, adults, children*

Generic name: Magnesium (sulfate, citrate, or hydroxide), castor oil *or* sodium phosphate

Dose: See label

Brand names: (Liquids) Adlerika, Alphamul, Castor Oil, Citrate of Magnesia, Citroma, Citro-Nesia, Concentrated Milk of Magnesia, Epsom Salt, Haley's M-O, Milk of Magnesia, Sodium Phosphates Oral Solution

Reasons: These agents all act very fast and differences are hard to identify. On the basis of taste, smell, or consistency, one may suit you more than another, but in terms of effectiveness, they are pretty equal.

Cautions: The nature of these agents and the way they work naturally leads to a greater incidence of unpleasant side effects. They stimulate bowel activity directly and may result in significant cramping and abdominal pain. However, if fast action is desired, these are the agents of choice. Repeated or frequent use is strongly discouraged, because it may result in a significant deficiency of nutrients and salts by preventing the absorption of required vitamins and minerals.

Constipation (Combination Laxatives for Oral Use) Intermediate Onset, Longer Duration

FIRST CHOICE

Generic name: Psyllium, senna, magnesium citrate, carboxy-methylcellulose, bisacodyl, casanthranol, *or* phenolphthalein

Dose: See label

Capsules: Disolan Forte, Evac-Q-Kit, Evac-Q-Kwik, Inner-clean Herbal Laxative

Liquids: Evac-Q-Kit, Evac-Q-Kwik

Reasons: These combination agents are designed to have an intermediate effect and a prolonged duration of effect. However, due to individual differences, they are not always successful. In most cases, the underlying problem needs to be resolved through adjustments in lifestyle or habits rather than use of laxatives. If short-term changes in routine (such as traveling) result in constipation, such agents may be useful to foster some regularity over a few days.

Cautions: When combinations of drugs are used, the ultimate effects are difficult to predict, due to the different ingredients used and the normal variability in response to drugs by different people. These agents may induce the typical symptoms of cramps or pain and perhaps diarrhea, or may be well tolerated.

Constipation (Suppositories) Fast Onset of Effect

FIRST CHOICE *for seniors, adults, children*

Generic name: Senna *or* bisacodyl *or* glycerin

Dose: Senna, 652 mg; bisacodyl, 10 mg; glycerin, see label

Brand names: Bisacodyl, Bisco-Lax, Dacodyl, Ducolax, Evac-Q-Kwik, Fleet Bisacodyl, Glycerin-USP, Sani-Supp, Senokot

Reasons: The direct effects of these agents on the bowel and the local application to the bowel by means of a suppository generally results in very satisfactory results and low side effects. In many cases they are preferred, but of course they are much less convenient and esthetically desirable, since the suppository must be inserted into the rectum.

Cautions: Due to the local nature of application and effect of these products, side effects are quite infrequent and there are no special problems to watch for.

Constipation (Enemas) Fast Onset of Effect

FIRST CHOICE *for seniors, adults, children*

Generic name: Glycerin, sodium phosphates, liquid castile soap, bisacodyl *or* mineral oil

Dose: See label

Brand names: Fleet Bagenema, Fleet Bagenema #1105, Fleet Bisacodyl, Fleet Enema, Fleet Mineral Oil, Fleet Pediatric Enema, Therac Plus, Therac-SB

Reasons: These products have several advantages due to the fact that they are given locally and act locally on the bowel. In addition, since they are given in liquid form, they supply one of the most important ingredients necessary to relieve constipation, water, to soften the stool. However, as mentioned for the suppositories, they are inconvenient to use and esthetically less desirable since they are administered into the rectum and may act almost immediately.

Cautions: These agents are designed to cause a rapid, complete evacuation of the bowels. Diarrhea may result and the side effects of cramping and abdominal pain may be very unpleasant. Loss of essential nutrients is part of the effect and repeated use is harmful. Follow label directions carefully.

Dehydration

Dehydration is a common result of persistent diarrhea or vomiting and during illness when the intake of food and liquids is not adequate. During all types of acute illness, drinking water or other clear liquids is very important to maintain proper water balance. The need for water may be increased by fever, and the reduced intake of food also reduces the total fluid intake. Salt and other minerals (electrolytes) may also become unbalanced when fluid or food intake is decreased, when diarrhea or vomiting occur, or in the presence of illness where increased losses of water occur (including a hangover, where alcohol has stimulated the kidneys to secrete extra water). To rehydrate, plain water or clear liquids are usually best; but in the special cases of diarrhea or vomiting, restoration of a proper fluid and electrolyte balance will be facilitated by using special formulations containing the most needed electrolytes. This is particularly true for children after a few days of diarrhea.

Rehydration Therapy

FIRST CHOICE

Brand names: Gatorade, Pedialyte (flavored or plain), Rehydralyte, Ricelyte

Reasons: The state of dehydration (not enough water in the body), and the loss of salts, buffers, and minerals from diarrhea or vomiting can prolong the illness and produce symptoms of fever, headache, nausea, and vomiting. Electrolyte solutions provide the various nutrients and extra calories to help restore energy and proper organ functions.

Cautions: These products are for use as supplements and aids to restore fluid and electrolyte balance during diarrhea or vomiting (when solid foods won't stay down) and do not provide all of the calorie or nutrient requirements. As soon as possible, solid foods and a balanced diet should be reinstituted. Severe deficiencies in fluid or electrolyte balance must be corrected rapidly. Consult your physician, especially for infants or small children, if diarrhea or vomiting is very severe or prolonged.

Hangover

A hangover is the result of overindulgence in alcohol. No specific highly effective agents are available, but home remedies are numerous for treatment of this problem. Because many of the symptoms result from the direct effects of alcohol, there are very few specific measures that are helpful. The first thing to do is to be sure to drink plenty of liquids, since one of the biggest problems is dehydration, a consequence of the diuretic effects of alcohol. For other symptoms, taking an antacid, an analgesic, and a stimulant (caffeine) have been shown to be of benefit and safe for treatment. Individual agents recommended are described below.

Hangover (Oral Use, Relief of Symptoms Only)
Individual Agents

FIRST CHOICE *for all groups*

Analgesic: Ibuprofen (see Chapter 2, page 21)

Antacid: Combination of aluminum and magnesium hydroxides (see page 92)

Stimulant: Caffeine (see Chapter 8, page 177)

Combination agents are available that combine other analgesics (aspirin or acetaminophen) and the stimulant (caffeine) for added convenience (see below). There are also several combination agents that combine the analgesic and an antacid. So far no agents containing all three of the symptom-reducing agents are on the market.

Hangover (Oral Use, Relief of Symptoms Only)
Combination Products

SECOND CHOICE

Analgesic with stimulant: Anacin, Maximum Strength Anacin, Excedrin Extra Strength, Aspirin Free Excedrin

Antacids: Excedrin Dual is a new product for headache and stomach upset containing acetaminophen and antacid (see page 83 for other choices).

Hiccups

Hiccups are a common and usually transient malady. Occasionally they may persist longer than an hour and eventually result in fatigue and incapacitation. There are no effective over-the-counter drugs for this disorder, but there are many home remedies that are widely touted as effective. None has been objectively tested or proven effective. Medical intervention may be helpful if a precipitating cause can be identified and treated. Several drugs have been used in a few instances and shown to be effective, but this may vary with the patient.

Various causes have been associated with hiccups, including excessive food or alcohol intake and sudden changes in temperature. Treatment of hiccups is more art than science. No drug is universally effective, nor are the myriad home remedies. Among the more successful measures are gargling with water, sipping ice water, swallowing granulated sugar, and biting on a lemon. Perhaps the best known is breathing into a paper bag. No firm advice can be given for this affliction; just try one or two and chances are they will go away.

Pinworms

Pinworms are small round worms that commonly infect humans, particularly children. They live in the intestine, but lay eggs on the skin just outside of the anus, which induces intense itching, the usual symptom that causes recognition of the infection. Scratching causes the irritation to be worse and may result in a secondary infection. The "Scotch tape" technique is most satisfactory for diagnosing the infection, by recovering the eggs (in the morning before a bowel movement or bath) around the anal opening. All infected individuals in the home must be treated simultaneously or the infection will reoccur. Exposure at school, on the playground, and so forth may also result in reinfections. Treatment failures are rare if the instructions are followed and measures taken to prevent reexposure to other infected individuals.

Anti-Worm Medicine

Pyrantel. Pyrantel is a good, broad spectrum, antihelmintic (worm-killing) drug in use for 20 years. It is effective and has very low toxicity, so it is available over the counter for use in pinworm infestations. It is taken by mouth, but mainly has a local effect in the intestine, since it is not absorbed very well. **Pregnant women:** Should not be used during pregnancy. **Nursing mothers:** no data. **Seniors:** no special problems. **Drug interactions:** none reported.

Pinworms (Oral Use)

FIRST (ONLY) CHOICE

Generic name: Pyrantel

Dose: 250 mg/ml

Brand names: Antiminth, Reese's Pinworm

Reasons: Pyrantel is very effective and quite safe, and the only agent available for use in this class.

Cautions: Pregnant women and anyone with liver disease should not use this drug. Sometimes intestinal upset occurs, and occasional headache or dizziness are noted. These side effects do not persist and are generally not severe enough to require treatment.

Stool Softeners

Stool softeners are used alone or in preparations to treat constipation and hemorrhoids. See pages 92–104 for full coverage of these problems.

Ingredients for Stool Softeners

Docusate. This ingredient has minimal laxative effects of its own, but is widely used as a stool softener. It is very useful to maintain a moist stool and prevent straining to have a bowel movement. This is particularly important in treating hemorrhoids and for anyone who has frequent problems with constipation. It is not effective until one to three days after administration. It interacts with some of the laxatives (especially the stimulant types).

Stool Softeners

FIRST CHOICE

Generic name: Docusate

Dose: 60–240 mg

Brand names: Afko-Lube (capsule and syrup), DC 240, Dialose, Diocto, Diocto-K, Dioctolose, Dioeze, Dio-Sul, Disonate (capsule, liquid, syrup), DOK, Doss, Duosol, D-S-S, Genasoft, Kasof, Laxinate, Liqui-Doss, Modane Soft, Pro-Cal-Sof, Pro-Sof, Regulax SS, Regutol, Softenex, Sulfalax, Surfak

Reasons: This is a safe and effective means of softening the stool.

Cautions: None of any consequence.

6

Skin Disorders

See Chapter 2 for oral products for burns, insect stings and bites, and fever associated with blisters and sores.

Numerous symptoms, diseases, and stresses affect the skin. Covering our entire body, it is subjected to a wide variety of insults and potential problems. Some of the problems arise from within and are expressed through the skin (like some allergies). Others are a direct result of a hostile environment attacking the surface, like fungal infections (athlete's foot), sunburn, poison ivy/oak/sumac, or just wear and tear (corns/calluses). There are many products to choose from and some are very effective for their intended purpose. This group of drugs contains many over-the-counter products that can actually cure problems rather than just treat symptoms. Each section is prefaced by a description of the particular problem and how to treat it effectively.

Acne

A common—almost universal—problem of adolescence, acne cannot be cured, but it can be treated very effectively with over-the-counter products. In many mild cases it can be cleared up completely. There are several products which, when used appropriately, can dramatically improve acne. In fact, most treatment failures have been found to be the result of improper use of these medications. The best ingredient in this class is *benzoyl peroxide*. It reduces both inflamed and noninflamed acne lesions, and when used correctly will prevent the development of new pimples. It must be used over the entire affected area; and, for optimal results, the time it is allowed to remain on the skin should be gradually increased daily (by about 30 minutes) until 8–10 hours total treatment time is attained.

Although other products, including antibiotics and antiseptics or abrasives, can be added or used instead, there is little evidence that they are any better than benzoyl peroxide, when it is used correctly. Corticosteroid-containing creams and lotions may also be used to reduce inflammation. There is some concern that benzoyl peroxide appears to increase certain tumors in mice, so alternative ingredients are listed for those who want to avoid even the slightest suggestion of risk. Most experts are confident that the increased tumors in mice do not suggest any increased risk of cancer for humans.

There is no scientific evidence that foods (including chocolate, nuts, cola drinks, potato chips, french fries, or other junk food) cause acne or make it worse. If you find that there is a food that triggers your acne, avoid it. In addition to puberty, the main factors that make acne worse are bacteria, dirt, oil, stress, menstruation, and some cosmetics. Generally, you should not pick at blemishes (pimples). You can make them worse by getting them infected or causing more damage to the skin.

Best Ingredients for Acne Treatment

Benzoyl peroxide. This agent was introduced in 1931 for the topical treatment of acne. It is available in several products at varying concentrations. Benzoyl peroxide works by removing the top layer of skin and helping to unblock the glands in the skin that get plugged and inflamed, causing comedones (blackheads, whiteheads, pimples). It can also reduce inflammation by killing bacteria that infects hair follicles. It is often irritating when first used, so tolerance must be built up gradually by slowly increasing the amount of time it is left on the skin each day. **Pregnant women:** safety not established. **Nursing mothers:** no evidence of risk. **Seniors:** not needed in this population. **Drug interactions:** topical use means low risk—none reported.

Sulfur. This agent is a mild fungicide and germicide and also acts to remove the top layer of skin as described above for benzoyl peroxide. It is generally milder than benzoyl peroxide, so it is a good choice for those with very sensitive skin or if you cannot build up tolerance to benzoyl peroxide through graduated use as directed. Sulfur works better when combined with salicylic acid, so this combination is the recommended choice as an alternative to benzoyl peroxide. **Pregnant women:** no evidence of risk. **Nursing mothers:** no evidence of risk. **Seniors:** not needed in this population. **Drug interactions:** topical use means low risk—none reported.

Salicylic acid. A derivative of aspirin, this agent has pronounced properties to remove a layer of skin cells. It is used topically for this purpose to treat acne, and also in higher concentrations for wart and corn or callus removal and similar uses. For treatment of acne, it is more effective when combined with sulfur. This combination is the second choice recommendation for treating acne. **Pregnant women:** no evidence of risk. **Nursing mothers:** no evidence of risk. **Seniors:** not needed in this population. **Drug interactions:** topical use means low risk—none reported.

Acne (Topical Therapy)

FIRST CHOICE *for adults, children*

Generic name: Benzoyl peroxide

Dose: 10% conc. (5% for sensitive skin)

Brand names: Acne-Aid, Ben-Aqua 10, Benoxyl 10, Clearasil Benzoyl Peroxide, Del-Aqua 10, Dry and Clear, Fostex 10% BPO, Noxzema Clear-Ups Acne Medicated Max Strength, Oxy 10, pHisoAc BP, Stri-Dex Maximum Strength, Xerac BP 10

Reasons: Benzoyl peroxide is the most effective medication available without a prescription for the treatment of acne. When used correctly, these agents are very effective for almost everyone. Follow directions carefully to obtain the best results and to minimize the most frequent side effects (dry, irritated skin).

Cautions: Irritation is a frequent side effect, and drying or stinging of the skin may also occur. By using a small amount and a short time of exposure, and gradually building up tolerance over several days, the drug will prove to be very effective for most acne sufferers.

Acne (Topical Therapy)

SECOND CHOICE *for adults, children*

Generic name: Sulfur *or* combination of sulfur (2–4%) plus salicylic acid (1–2%)

Dose: Sulfur alone, 8% conc.; in combination, sulfur, 2–4% and salicylic acid, 1–2%

Brand names: Acnomel, Acnotex, Bensulfoid, Clearasil Adult Care, Pernox Lotion, Sebasorb, Therac

Reasons: Sulfur and salicylic acid are less effective than benzoyl peroxide, the first choice. However, they do have a role, particularly for individuals who are sensitive to the irritation caused by benzoyl peroxide.

Cautions: These topical agents are quite safe and only infrequently cause the problems usually associated with topical therapy, including irritation, redness, or stinging of the skin at the sites of application.

Allergic Skin Reactions

Numerous different types of skin rashes can be caused by allergic reactions to various chemicals, plants, foods, drugs, or almost anything else that may contact the skin. It is often difficult to determine the cause of a rash. Even experts must often resort to sophisticated tests or even trial-and-error testing to find the source of the problem and an effective treatment. When the rash occurs very quickly after contact, it is fairly easy to diagnose. However, in many cases, the rash takes hours or a day or two before it appears, and the connection to the agent contacting the skin and inducing the response is easily overlooked.

Rashes caused by ingestion or inhalation of offending allergens are much harder to pin down accurately. Hives is a type of rash that appears quickly and forms "bubbles" of swelling that are usually very pale in color and often surrounded by red outlines. They may be of any size and may combine, or "grow" as the reaction develops. Itching is often the first sign. The rash usually remains at a site for a few hours. Other types of rashes are more difficult to recognize. Among the most common are the "contact" reactions to poison ivy, poison oak, and poison sumac; but these reactions also occur after exposure to many other chemicals and products that contact the skin. In some cases the rash is due to an infection (yeast, bacteria, fungi, for example). If the cause can be determined, the treatment can be more specific (see other subjects as listed). If not, some general symptomatic relief can be provided with the agents described below.

Ingredients for Allergic Skin Rashes

Anti-inflammatory: hydrocortisone. This drug is actually a hormone produced naturally by the body. Used topically to relieve itch and irritation, it has potent anti-inflammatory effects. It is effectively used in a wide variety of other diseases and provides relief from several different symptoms. Overuse may lead to permanent thinning of the skin, as well as other more serious (but rare) adverse effects (altered mineral and fat metabolism). When used as directed it is one of the safest and is the best product for treating allergic skin rashes. **Pregnant women:** no evidence of risk. **Nursing mothers:** passes into breast milk. **Seniors:** no special problems, but decreased dose desirable if used often to reduce possible side effects on skin. **Drug interactions:** topical use means low risk.

Antihistamine: diphenhydramine. One of the oldest and most widely used antihistamines, this drug can be applied topically and may provide some additional relief for itching and redness by blocking the effects of histamine. However, many authorities feel this effect is of no real value and have called for the removal of topical antihistamines from the marketplace. Diphenhydramine is recognized as very safe, but when applied topically it may occasionally lead to development of a contact allergic reaction to the drug. **Pregnant women:** no evidence of risk. **Nursing mothers:** passes into the breast milk. **Seniors:** decrease dose to reduce side effects. **Drug interactions:** topical use means low risk—none reported.

Astringents: calamine or zinc oxide. These agents act on the skin's surface to protect and soften diseased or damaged layers of skin. They are soothing and help to reduce itching and irritation. There are many related drugs and some distinctions between their effects can be made, but superiority overall is hard to establish. These agents are recommended for topical application to soothe and relieve irritation caused by skin rashes, insect stings or bites, poison ivy/oak/sumac, and other related skin problems. **Pregnant women:** no evidence of risk. **Nursing mothers:** no evidence of risk. **Seniors:** no special problems. **Drug interactions:** topical use means low risk—none reported.

Local anesthetic: benzocaine. Introduced 85 years ago, benzocaine is one of the first local anesthetics. It is used in many diverse formulations for surface pain relief and also for itching. It is very poorly absorbed through the skin or mucous membranes, which makes it quite safe for use. It has few adverse effects, though occasionally a person may become allergic to it. **Pregnant women:** no evidence of risk. **Nursing mothers:** no evidence of risk. **Seniors:** no special problems. **Drug interactions:** topical use means very low risk.

Local anesthetic: lidocaine. Lidocaine has a rapid onset of effect, more penetrating ability, and a longer duration of effect (about one hour) than benzocaine. It is widely available in different products for pain and itching. Used for over 40 years, it is also quite safe and effective. **Pregnant women:** no evidence of risk. **Nursing mothers:** no evidence of risk. **Seniors:** no special problems. **Drug interactions:** topical use means low risk—none reported.

Local anesthetic: dibucaine. Dibucaine is a very potent local anesthetic with quite long-lasting effects. Due to these properties, it also has a somewhat higher incidence of side effects (headache, dizziness). It is most useful for prolonged relief and when the maximum anesthetic effect is desired. **Pregnant women:** no evidence of risk. **Nursing mothers:** no evidence of risk. **Seniors:** no special problems. **Drug interactions:** topical use means very low risk—none reported.

Allergy/Skin Rash (Topical Anti-inflammatory Effects)

FIRST CHOICE *for seniors, adults, children*

Generic name: Hydrocortisone

Dose: 0.5–1% conc.

Creams: Anusol HC-1, Bactine, CaldeCORT, Cortaid, Cortizone-5, Dermacort, Dermolate, Dermtex HC, Foille-Cort, H2 Cort, Hydrocortisone, Hydro-Tex, Hytone, Lanacort, Pharmacort, Preparation HC, Racet SE, Rhulicort

Lotions: Cortaid, Delacort, Dermacort, Hydrocortisone, Rhulicort

Ointments: Cortaid, Cortizone-5

Sprays: Cortaid

Reasons: Hydrocortisone is clearly the best overall topical treatment for skin rashes and inflammation of many types, particularly allergic reactions. Initially, it is best when used three times a day for a faster onset of effect. After the first day or two, using it once a day is probably just as effective as more frequent use. For dry, scaly eczema-type skin rashes, a greasy (ointment) formulation is best. For oozing or crusty lesions the cream formulations are superior. The lotions are less greasy, and the spray-on product is easy to use.

Cautions: Excessive use of hydrocortisone preparations can lead to problems locally or, in extreme cases, even to general toxic effects if too much is absorbed. Thinning of the skin (which can be permanent) is the most serious problem, and some increased susceptibility to infection (especially if the skin is broken) may result. When used as directed on the label, these products are some of the safest and most effective agents available for over-the-counter use.

Allergy/Skin Rash (Topical Use, Combination Drugs)

SECOND CHOICE *for seniors, adults, children*

Generic name: Diphenhydramine (antihistamine) *with* calamine or zinc oxide (astringent) *and* benzocaine (anesthetic)

Dose: See label

Brand names: Caladryl, Calamatum, Dalicote, Ivarest, Poison Ivy Spray, Rhuli Cream, Rhuli Spray, Ziradryl

Reasons: Little information is available on this class of agents as far as the true benefit of their use or comparison of different products. They can provide symptomatic relief and reduce the irritation, itching, and discomfort, which allows the healing process to proceed.

Cautions: Because these products are applied topically and are not absorbed into the system (blood), they have virtually no toxicity of consequence. Rarely, someone may develop an allergic reaction to one of the ingredients, and the use of the product will cause a rash and itching. Since these are usually the symptoms being treated, such side effects are difficult to recognize.

Bacterial Infections

There are two classes of drugs for treating bacterial infections: antibiotics and antiseptics. Antibiotics cannot be used orally without a prescription, but several topical agents are available over the counter. Unfortunately, they are not highly effective. They do not penetrate very far into the skin, and they may induce allergic reactions in some individuals, especially when they are used repeatedly. However, for minor infections or to help prevent infection after minor wounds, they can be useful.

Only minor skin infections should be self-treated. Most of the effort in this area is directed at preventing the development of infections. When the skin is damaged, washing with soap and water is important to clean the wound. Antiseptics (which kill bacteria) may then be applied to reduce the possibility of infection. Most are not very effective or are of very limited duration (see page 122). Antibiotic creams may also be used. Although not necessary in most cases, they provide some peace of mind and they can provide some benefit by hastening healing. Studies to evaluate the usefulness of prophylactic (preventive) antibiotic use, or even the use of antiseptics, have not provided clear-cut answers. The benefit is apparently small, but the use of such agents may reduce infections, particularly if the injury occurred outdoors, was due to broken glass, or resulted in an exposure to bacteria. Proper cleaning, or even soaking in warm saline (salt water), seems to be as effective as antibiotic or antiseptic treatment in most cases, however. The wound should be kept covered and in a humid environment, while allowing air access. It should also be insulated from hot or cold extremes and protected from secondary infection using bandages. Complete healing requires about two weeks.

Antiseptics are chemicals that have the ability to kill bacteria (and sometimes other germs as well) and cause only minimal irritation to the skin. There are a rather large number of products, and making comparisons is difficult due to the limited amount of testing done with these agents. *Alcohol, iodine, hydrogen peroxide,* and many more are available in a wide range of products. The usefulness of such agents is limited, and only a few will be discussed in this section.

Antibiotic Ingredients for
Bacterial Infections

Polymyxin B. Polymixin B is a bactericidal agent (one that kills bacteria) that is active on the surface to prevent or cure infections. It is not absorbed, reducing the possibility of side effects but limiting its effect. Resistance of the bacteria to this drug is very rare, making it very useful and effective in that regard. **Pregnant women:** no evidence of risk. **Nursing mothers:** no evidence of risk. **Seniors:** no special problems. **Drug interactions:** topical use means low risk—none reported.

Bacitracin. Used since 1948, bacitracin is an antibiotic that acts by a different mechanism and on a different group of bacteria than the polymyxin B described above. It is also for topical use and has a very low incidence of side effects (rarely an allergic reaction may develop). It is commonly used in combination with other agents to provide a very broad antibacterial effect. **Pregnant women:** no evidence of risk. **Nursing mothers:** no evidence of risk. **Seniors:** no special problems. **Drug interactions:** topical use means low risk—none reported.

Neomycin sulfate. Another long-used agent, this is a broad spectrum antibiotic (meaning it is effective against many different germs). It is also very effective and safe for topical use, although of all the agents in this group, it probably has the most likelihood of inducing an allergic reaction in the skin. **Pregnant women:** no evidence of risk. **Nursing mothers:** no evidence of risk. **Seniors:** no special problems. **Drug interactions:** topical use means low risk—none reported.

Tetracycline. Tetracycline is a broad spectrum bacteriostatic agent (meaning it stops bacterial growth), effective against a wide variety of bacteria (often used for acne). Although it is not used as frequently as the combination of the other agents described previously, it is a good alternative if there should be any irritation or allergy to the widely used triple combination of first choice. **Pregnant women:** no evidence of risk for topical use. **Nursing mothers:** no evidence of risk. **Seniors:** no special problems. **Drug interactions:** topical use means low risk—none reported.

Topical Antibiotics

FIRST CHOICE *for seniors, adults, children*

Generic name: Polymyxin B *and* bacitracin *and* neomycin sulfate

Dose: See label

Brand names: Bactine First Aid Antibiotic, Lanabiotic Ointment, Medi-Quik, Mycitracin, N.B.P., Neomixin, Neosporin, Neo-Thrycex, Septa, Trimycin, Triple Antibiotic

Reasons: The combination of polymyxin B, bacitracin, and neomycin sulfate gives the broadest possible coverage of anti-infective potential. Each of the three has a different spectrum of germs that it kills and when the three are combined, the prophylactic (preventive) effect, or the ability to effect a cure of surface infections, is maximized.

Cautions: As with nearly all topically applied drugs, the main potential side effect is the development of an allergic reaction. This problem is fairly minor, and the number of people that become allergic is small but must be considered if the infection is not cured quickly, or the site remains (or becomes) irritated after a few days of use.

Topical Antibiotics

SECOND CHOICE *for seniors, adults, children*

Generic name: Tetracycline *or* single/double mixture from triple combination first choice (described above)

Dose: See label

Brand names: Acromycin, Aureomycin, Baciguent, Bacitracin, Myciguent, Neomycin, Neosporin Cream, Polysporin (ointment and powder), Terramycin

Reasons: The single agent, or combination of two, does not have as broad a spectrum of antibiotic activity as the first choice, but these products are a good alternative if for some reason the first choice is not effective, or you are allergic to one of the three antibiotics used in the first choice products.

Cautions: There are few adverse effects from the use of these agents topically. The occasional development of an allergic reaction is about the only side effect to watch for. These reactions are not serious and by discontinuing use of the drug, the rash or irritation will go away.

Antiseptic Ingredients for Bacterial Infections

Iodine. Iodine is one of the more effective antiseptics and comes in several different forms. Perhaps the best is iodine tincture, which is iodine in alcohol, but it burns like fire. Iodine solution stings less and is less effective. **Pregnant women:** no evidence of risk. **Nursing mothers:** no evidence of risk. **Seniors:** no special problems. **Drug interactions:** topical use means low risk—none reported.

Hydrogen peroxide. Hydrogen peroxide is an old, effective antiseptic. It works well, but its effect is of very brief duration. This is one of the natural products the body makes and uses to kill germs. **Pregnant women:** no evidence of risk. **Nursing mothers:** no evidence of risk. **Seniors:** no special problems. **Drug interactions:** topical use means low risk—none reported.

Benzalkonium chloride. This is the most commonly used drug in this class and is a fairly good antiseptic. A major limitation is that it is destroyed by soap. If the wound is washed and then rinsed very well, and no soap remains, then it will be helpful when applied. But if soap is left behind, it will do nothing. **Pregnant women:** no evidence of risk. **Nursing mothers:** no evidence of risk. **Seniors:** no special problems. **Drug interactions:** topical use means low risk—none reported.

Topical Antiseptics

FIRST CHOICE *for adults, children*

Generic name: Benzalkonium chloride

Dose: See label

Brand names: Bactine, Benzalkonium Chloride, Zephiran Chloride Solution and Spray

Reasons: These products all contain the first choice antiseptic ingredient, which has a fairly broad spectrum of antimicrobial effectiveness and is quite safe. They can be used to clean wounds and dramatically reduce the germ count to reduce the possibility of infection. If any soap remains on the skin after washing, this antiseptic will not work.

Cautions: There are few side effects associated with this agent, and none of concern. Used as directed, it is safe and useful for its intended purpose.

Topical Antiseptics

SECOND CHOICE *for adults, children*

Generic name: Iodine

Dose: See label

Brand names: ACU-dyne, Biodyne Topical 1%, Efodine, Iodex Regular, Iodine Strong Solution

Reasons: Iodine has been used for many years to disinfect and clean wounds to prevent infections. It is quite safe and useful for this purpose. It is the second choice mainly because of the possibility of staining clothing and in some formulations, because of the stinging it causes.

Cautions: Iodine is also quite safe and should present no problems when used as directed on the product package.

Burns

Each year 1 in every 100 Americans seeks medical attention for burns. The incidence in children is particularly high, especially from scalds with hot liquids. Depending on the severity, burns can cause many problems, from fluid, salt, and metabolism problems, to infections and functional impairment. Most burns are minor, but each must be carefully assessed to be sure that more serious damage was not done than is at first apparent.

Electrical burns at home (110 volts) may cause heart irregularities, but burns from higher voltages (220 volts or more) can cause deep tissue injuries that cannot be seen and should be referred to an expert. In general, only first-degree burns should be self-treated. A first-degree burn is where the burn is confined to the superficial skin, which becomes red and then turns white (blanches) when pressure is applied. This is most often the result of sun exposure, very short flashes of fire, or short exposure to moderately hot liquids. If blisters form or loss of sensation occurs, medical care is required to evaluate the seriousness of the burn and to determine the appropriate treatment. To care for burns, the source of the burn must first be immediately removed and any clothing removed from the site. Cool water should be applied for up to three hours after the burn occurs to decrease the heat and pain. Oral analgesics should also be administered as soon as possible (see Chapter 2, page 21), and topical analgesics may be used for defined areas to help relieve the pain (see Chapter 2, page 44). Antihistamines may be useful after a few days to help reduce the itching that accompanies the healing process (see Chapter 4, page 69).

The best drugs for first-degree burns are the local anesthetics: benzocaine, lidocaine, and dibucaine. You can use the same drugs for effective relief from the itching and pain associated with bites, stings, and poison ivy/oak/and sumac. For more about the rash from these plants, see page 144.

Burns, Bites/Stings, Itching, Pain (Topical Treatment, Pain Relief Only)

FIRST CHOICE *for seniors, adults, children*

Generic name: Benzocaine

Dose: 10–20% conc. (spray), 5–10% (cream, lotion)

Aerosols: aeroCaine, aeroTherm, Americaine, Burntame, Dermoplast, Lanacaine, Solarcaine, Sting Relief, Tega Caine

Creams/lotions: Americaine, Benzocaine, Benzocol, Bicozene, Dermoplast, Foille, Lagol, Medicone Dressing, Solarcaine, Sting Kill (swabs), Sting Relief

Reasons: Benzocaine is the best overall local anesthetic for topical use, having a good balance of effect, duration of action, and safety. Some of the others are more potent or last longer, but have more toxicity, so products containing benzocaine are overall the best choice.

Cautions: These have the lowest potential for side effects of all the alternatives for this treatment group.

Burns, Bites/Stings, Itching, Pain (Topical Treatment, Pain Relief Only)

SECOND CHOICE *for seniors, adults, children*

Generic name: Lidocaine *or* dibucaine

Dose: Lidocaine, 1–2.5% conc.; *or* dibucaine, 0.5%–1% conc.

Brand names: After Burn Plus (gel and spray), Bactine First Aid (aerosol and liquid), Dibucaine (ointment), Medi-Quik (spray), Nupercainal (cream), Solarcaine (cream, lotion), Unguentine Plus (cream), Xylocaine (ointment)

Reasons: These two alternatives for local anesthetic effect are both more potent and longer lasting than the first choice noted above (benzocaine). However, they seem to be somewhat less effective overall, particularly for this type of relief, and they have more toxic potential than benzocaine, so remain the second choice.

Cautions: Due to possible side effects, follow label directions regarding the amount and timing of reapplication. If skin irritation occurs, discontinue use immediately.

Cold/Canker Sores and Fever Blisters

Sores on the lips or in the mouth are usually caused by viruses and are a recurring problem in 20–45% of the general population. These sores recur randomly throughout life. Pain and discomfort are the most common symptoms, but are usually resolved, or at least decrease, within a day or two. The sores normally require about eight days to heal. Relief of symptoms is the primary treatment, but the size of the lesion may also be reduced and the pain lessened by the very early application of the agents described in this section. As soon as the earliest sign of a developing sore (tingling or itching) is noted, the medication should be applied. For relief of pain from an established sore, the second choice agents are topical anesthetics (pain relievers).

Ingredients for Treatment of Lip Sores

Tannic acid. When applied topically, tannic acid has properties that kill some viruses. There are few therapeutic uses for it aside from treating viral sores on the lips. It can be toxic to the liver if too much is taken internally.

Salicylic acid. This agent is a derivative of aspirin. It is effective due to its properties to remove a layer(s) of skin cells. It may cause irritation of the surrounding skin, so apply it carefully to the intended area to minimize irritation.

Carbamide peroxide. Simular to the combination of the two ingredients described above (salicylic acid and tannic acid) in its properties, but milder. This ingredient is also available pending a final decision from the USFDA on whether it is safe and effective for canker sore treatment. It is approved for earwax removal.

Cold/Canker Sores and Fever Blisters (Topical Treatment to Reduce Size)

FIRST CHOICE *for seniors, adults, children*

Generic name: Tannic acid *and* salicylic acid

Dose: Tannic acid, 7% conc.; salicylic acid, 2.5% conc.

Brand names: Zilactol. (Several other brands contain tannic acid with benzocaine, but it's not clear if they also reduce sore size. Examples: Orajel CSM, Orasept Liquid, Tanac)

Reasons: Although the USFDA (U. S. Food and Drug Administration) has not yet ruled whether tannic acid is effective, a recent clinical trial showed a clear benefit in reducing the size of the sores when it was applied soon after the first symptoms were noted.

Cautions: These agents are safe, especially since they are used topically. They should not be ingested and should be applied directly on the sore to minimize irritation effects.

Cold/Canker Sores and Fever Blisters (Topical Treatment for Pain Relief Only)

SECOND CHOICE *for seniors, adults, children*

Generic name: Benzocaine *or* carbamide peroxide

Dose: Benzocaine 15–20% conc. *or* 10% carbamide peroxide

Brand names: Anbesol Maximum Strength (gel and liquid), Benzodent, Cankaid, Gly-oxide, Kank-A Liquid Professional Strength, Orabase (B or O), Orajel Maximum Strength, Orajel Mouth Aid, Proxigel

Reasons: Benzocaine is the best overall local anesthetic for topical use, having a good balance of effect, duration, and safety. Some of the other local anasthetics are more potent or last longer but have more toxicity, so products containing benzocaine are overall the best choice.

Cautions: Benzocaine has the lowest potential for side effects of all the alternatives for this treatment group.

Corns and Calluses

These common skin afflictions result from the repeated trauma of pressure or friction to the skin, often over joints or between digits. This problem is frequent in a society that requires that shoes be worn, and where style is more important than comfort and practicality. The skin becomes very thick and painful as a result of the hardened, usually round, area of dry, dead skin that builds up as protection. Fungal infections may occur secondarily at the site. Prophylactic (preventive) treatment is most effective, by changing to soft shoes or using protective bandages of some sort to pad the area. The corn or callus may be removed with the preparations containing salicylic acid described below. A nail file or emery board may also be useful to reduce the size of the corn or callus and make removal easier and faster.

Active Ingredient for Corns and Calluses

Salicylic acid. This agent is a derivative of aspirin. It is effective due to its properties to remove a layer(s) of skin cells. It is used topically for this purpose to treat acne, and also in higher concentrations for wart, corn, and callus removal and similar uses. It may cause irritation of the surrounding skin, so apply carefully to the intended area to minimize irritation. **Pregnant women:** no evidence of risk. **Nursing mothers:** no evidence of risk. **Seniors:** no special problems. **Drug interactions:** topical use means low risk—none reported.

Corns and Calluses (Topical Treatment to Remove)

FIRST CHOICE *for seniors, adults, children*

Generic name: Salicylic acid

Dose: 20–40% conc.

Brand names: Dr. Scholl's Corn Removers (and Waterproof Corn Removers), Mosco

Reasons: These products use the highest concentrations of active ingredient and an occlusive dressing to help speed the effects. Other preparations using lower levels of active drug are less irritating, but may not be effective, or take considerably longer to work.

Cautions: These topically applied and fast-acting products are generally very safe. The only thing to watch for is irritation of the surrounding normal skin. By carefully limiting the application to the intended site, this problem is minimal.

Corns and Calluses (Topical Treatment to Remove)

SECOND CHOICE *for seniors, adults, children*

Generic name: Salicylic acid

Dose: 10–17% conc.

Brand names: Compound W Wart Remover, Dr. Scholl's Wart Remover, Gets-it Liquid, Off Ezy Wart Removal Kit, Wart-Off

Reasons: These products contain a lower concentration of the only active ingredient that is effective for corn and callus removal. They will probably work, but will require a longer treatment period. In some cases however, they may not be effective, and the higher concentration products listed under the first choice will be needed.

Cautions: The incidence of side effects with these agents is quite low. Again, the only thing to watch for is irritation of the surrounding normal skin.

Dandruff and Seborrhea

The latest information on both of these conditions is that they are caused by surface yeast infections. There are a number of agents for treatment of these conditions, and the only thing they have in common appears to be the ability to cure yeast infections. The association of yeast with these diseases has been noted for some time, but not recognized as the cause until recently. Dandruff is one of the most common dermatological (skin) problems—up to 70% of the population suffers from it—yet it has never been studied well. Several agents are quite effective and their use and the advantages of each will be described. See also, "Seborrhea," page 151, which has slightly different recommended treatments.

Best Ingredients for Dandruff

Selenium sulfide. This bright orange drug is the best over-the-counter agent for treating/preventing dandruff, as shown by comparison trials. Its effect is local, and it produces a complete cure in a large majority of cases after four weeks of use. Both the rate of cure and the percentage of individuals cured is higher for this ingredient than the others listed below. In addition to antifungal effects, it appears to reduce the turnover rate of the scalp skin to help reduce flakiness. It should be used only as often as needed to control dandruff. Watch for toxicity to the eyes (keep out of eyes), and orange tinting of gray hair is possible. **Pregnant women:** no evidence of risk. **Nursing mothers:** no evidence of risk. **Seniors:** no special problems. **Drug interactions:** topical use means low risk—none reported.

Zinc pyrithione. This agent comes in not too far behind selenium as an effective treatment for dandruff. It has antimicrobial activity and may also reduce skin turnover. The cure takes longer than with selenium, but this agent is less toxic than selenium. **Pregnant women:** no evidence of risk. **Nursing mothers:** no evidence of risk. **Seniors:** no special problems. **Drug interactions:** topical use means low risk—none reported.

Coal tar and salicylic acid. Either one of these agents can be used alone, but they are not terribly effective. However, as a team they have some antifungal activity and the ability to remove the dead skin where yeast lives. The appeal of these products is that the smell and side effects of their use tend to be lower than for the other agents in this class. If they are effective, you are in good shape. If not, you may have to resort to the more effective agents in this class. These products must be used for several weeks to be effective. **Pregnant women:** no evidence of risk. **Nursing mothers:**

Reasons: Very little toxicity or side effects are noted with is ingredient. It has antimicrobial activity and gradual improve-ent is noted in most patients over several weeks of use.

Cautions: None of special concern.

Dandruff (Topical Treatment to Clear It Up)

THIRD CHOICE *for seniors, adults, children*

Generic name: Coal tar and salicylic acid (some also with ulfur)

Dose: See label

Brand names: Fostex Medicated, Ionil T, Neutrogena T/Gel, Sebex-T, Tarsum, Tar Dandruff Shampoo, Vanseb-T, X-Seb

Reasons: This class of product is a combination agent, which is better than those containing either one of the single-agent products. It is generally well accepted by patients for reasons of smell, side effects, and the overall esthetics of use. It is less effective than the other choices, but may be preferred nonetheless. The anti-fungal activity of coal tar is minimal, which is why the combination is recommended. Used regularly, it will reduce dandruff.

Cautions: None of special concern.

Diaper Rash

Diaper rash is difficult to treat effectively because it varies so much among infants. The skin rash can be the result of direct effects of the bowel waste products (stool) burning the skin, or from bacte-rial, fungal, or yeast infections. The skin of infants and young chil-dren is thinner and less firm than adults. Factors often producing diaper rash include moisture retention by wet diapers and rubber pants, which causes skin to be inflamed; direct chemical effects of the products excreted in urine and stool; mechanical and chemical irritants (like too tight a diaper or pants); soap; and the occurrence of infections.

no evidence of risk. **Seniors:** no special problems. [...]
tions: topical use means low risk—none reported.

Dandruff (Topical Treatment to Clear It Up

FIRST CHOICE *for seniors, adults, children*

Generic name: Selenium sulfide

Dose: 1% conc.

Brand names: (shampoo or lotion) Selsun Blue,
Sulfide

Reasons: This agent is the most effective over-th
treatment for dandruff. It is not clear exactly how it w
several beneficial effects have been noted. Very little of th
absorbed, making it generally safe. After four weeks of t
two of every three people are cured. It also shows the fast
on dandruff of all the agents in this class.

Cautions: Take care to keep these products out of y
as this drug can have adverse effects. On continued use
leave a smell and make the hair oily. It may also cause ora
ing to gray hair.

Dandruff (Topical Treatment to Clear It Up)

SECOND CHOICE *for seniors, adults, children*

Generic name: Zinc pyrithione

Dose: 1–2% conc.

Shampoos: Anti-Dandruff Brylcreem, Breck One, D
DHS Zinc, Head & Shoulders, Sebex, Sebulon, Zincon

Creams/lotions: Breck One

To treat diaper rash, change the diapers frequently, wash the skin thoroughly using mild soap, rinse it well, and apply powder or an ointment to protect the skin as much as possible. Infections can be treated effectively with the proper medication. A note of caution—some practitioners recommend using a hair dryer to thoroughly dry the skin. This is *not* a good idea, since these appliances can expel very hot air after only a couple of minutes of use, producing significant burns very quickly. Since hot, humid conditions promote infections with fungi and yeast, it is best to dry the skin with a towel and apply powder or a protective ointment to protect the skin from excess moisture and the irritating waste products. The best agents are described in this section.

Recommended Skin Protectants

Petrolatum. Petrolatum is the best of the softener/moisturizer/protectant (emollient) ingredients for use on the skin for a variety of diseases and symptoms. This ointment (water in oil) serves to protect and shield the skin from external irritating substances by taking up water and forming an occlusive barrier to prevent the loss of water. An alternative is the animal fat derivative, *lanolin*, but because many people are or can become allergic to this wool-derived fat, it is not highly recommended for use. Other alternatives include *mineral oil* and various *vegetable oils* (like *cocoa butter*), but no clear advantages or additional arguments for their use over petrolatum have been proven. Pregnant women: no evidence of risk. **Nursing mothers:** no evidence of risk. **Seniors:** no special problems.

Zinc oxide. This is the best of several rather innocuous, inert substances used to help cover and protect the skin and membrane surfaces. It increases the smoothness and decreases friction and protects the skin, especially from sun and wind burn. *Talc* and *corn starch* also serve similar purposes, but become doughy when they absorb moisture. **Pregnant women:** no evidence of risk. **Nursing mothers:** no evidence of risk. **Seniors:** no special problems.

Diaper Rash—Skin Protectant (Topical Ointments)

FIRST CHOICE *for infants*

Generic name: Petrolatum *or* zinc oxide

Dose: See label

Brand names: A and D Ointment, Aveeno Oilated, Balmex, B-Balm Baby, Caldesene Medicated, Comfortine, Desitin, Vaseline Pure Petroleum Jelly

Reasons: Both petrolatum and zinc oxide are very good protectants. They act to retain moisture and keep irritating substances from contacting the skin. Some products contain additional ingredients that may add to their cost, but additional benefits have not been demonstrated.

Cautions: None of concern.

Diaper Rash—Powder (Without Medication)

FIRST CHOICE

Generic name: Petrolatum *or* zinc oxide *or* talc *or* oatmeal

Dose: See label

Brand names: Aveeno Colloidal Oatmeal, Balmex Baby, Johnson's Baby, ZBT Baby, Zeasorb

Reasons: All of the noted ingredients have useful, desired effects to help keep the skin dry and protect it from the moisture, waste products, and other irritations that can trigger or aggravate diaper rash. No good comparison testing has been published to allow meaningful distinctions to be made among the various products.

Cautions: The combination of topical application and long experience with their use makes these preparations very safe. No significant side effects are expected.

Diaper Rash—Antifungal (Topical Use)

FIRST CHOICE

Generic name: Tolnaftate *or* miconazole

Dose: 1–2% conc.

Brand names: Aftate, Dr. Scholl's Athlete's Foot Cream, Genaspor, Micatin, NP-27, Tinactin, Ting, Zeasorb-AF

Reasons: Although miconazole is more effective overall against fungal infections, both of the antifungal agents recommended here as first choice are very safe and are expected to cure diaper rash if it involves a fungal infection.

Cautions: These drugs are safe and only rarely produce adverse effects, including itching, irritation, or rash.

Diaper Rash—Antimicrobial (Topical, Bacterial Infections)

FIRST CHOICE

Generic name: Polymyxin B *and* bacitracin *and* neomycin sulfate

Dose: See label

Brand names: Bactine First Aid Antibiotic, Lanabiotic Ointment, Medi-Quik, Mycitracin, N.B.P., Neomixin, Neosporin, Neo-Thrycex, Septa, Trimycin, Triple Antibiotic

Reasons: Each of the three antibacterial agents kills different bacteria. The combination is used to ensure that the infection is cured.

Cautions: As with all combination agents, the risk of adverse effects is increased by having several drugs present. In this case, the topical application and nature of these drugs limit the possibilities of adverse effects to local irritation, redness, or rash, as a result of an allergic response developing to one of the ingredients. If this occurs, single agents may be substituted for the combination.

Dry Skin

Severely dry skin may be characterized by scaling, redness (erythema), cracking, itching, soreness, and tenderness. Many factors can influence the development of dry skin, which is due to loss of water (not oil) from the skin. Fair skin and advancing age are common predisposing factors, but excessive bathing; long exposure to low humidity, strong soaps, solvents, and ultraviolet light (sunshine); and swimming also contribute to the problem. To treat dry skin, you must do all you can to reduce the breakdown of the skin's natural protection (oils) and/or replenish this protection to limit water loss. Reduce your exposure to the contributing factors as much as possible.

Creams or lotions containing oil can also be very effective to treat dry skin. Creams contain more oil than lotions and are therefore generally superior. The best of all for dry skin, but usually unacceptable for cosmetic reasons (except perhaps at bedtime) are ointments like petroleum jelly or vegetable shortening. Products containing alcohol should be avoided, since alcohol causes drying. Mild soaps containing glycerin produce the least drying effects. Creams or lotions should be applied while the skin is moist. There are so many products that comparisons among them are impractical, so trial and error is about the only way to find what works for you. The products listed here have the highest recommendations and best ingredients to tackle this problem. For acute relief of itching and inflammation, the topical steroids are by far the most effective (see page 160).

Dry Skin Formulations

Ointments. A mixture of water in oil, these products maintain a greater amount of water in the skin, but are greasy, sticky, and often unacceptable for routine use. Twice-a-day use is usually sufficient, but use at bedtime is most desirable and least objectionable.

Creams. An emulsion of oil in water, creams can be very effective, depending on how much oil is incorporated into the product. They are best applied every four hours for maximum benefit.

Lotions. Lotions are a suspension of powder crystals dissolved in water. They have a cooling effect on the skin, but are less occlusive and provide less protection than creams and ointments. They are easier to apply and do not leave a greasy feeling. They must be applied quite frequently to be effective.

Gels. These are preparations containing alcohol as a base and therefore liquify on contact with the skin. They disappear quickly, but should not be used for dry skin because the alcohol itself has a drying effect and can cause burning of sensitive, irritated, dry skin.

Urea-containing products. Some dry skin products contain urea, which is thought to change skin cells to make them hold more water. These products are more expensive and probably not cost-effective for dry skin. A good cream is likely to offer all of the needed moisturizing effect when used properly, at less cost.

Dry Skin Treatment

FIRST CHOICE

Generic name: Petrolatum *or* mineral oil (products containing high levels of these)

Dose: See label

Ointments: Plexolan, Saratoga

Creams: Acid Mantel, Allercreme Ultra Emollient, Curel Moisturizing, Lanoline, Lubriderm, Moisturel, Purpose Dry Skin, Vaseline Dermatology Formula

Lotions: Allercreme Skin, Curel Moisturizing, Dermassage, Eclipse After Sun, Eucerin, Keri, Moisturel, Nivea Moisturizing, Nutraderm 30, Sofenol 5, Vaseline Dermatology Formula, Wondra

Reasons: These products contain the highest concentrations of the most effective ingredients for dry skin treatment. They effectively keep the moisture in the skin and prevent drying when used as directed.

Cautions: None of concern.

Fungal Infections

Athlete's foot, jock itch, some types of diaper rash, and ringworm are the result of fungi that grow on the skin in various locations. Fungal infections of the skin, scalp, and nails are probably second only to acne as the most frequent skin disease. The fungi do not live on living tissue, but only on the dead outer layer of the skin. They are not serious diseases, but can affect the quality of life, and are readily treated with very effective and safe over-the-counter agents.

These infections must be treated with good hygiene as well as antifungal agents to both cure them and prevent their return. You can reinfect yourself repeatedly from your shower, clothing, or shoes. Keep your feet and groin area clean and dry, since fungi loves a moist environment. Change socks, underwear, or jock strap often, and allow these areas to "breathe" as much as possible. Wash well with soap and water, but don't be too rough. Powder may be used to help dry these areas and keep them dry.

Ringworm is a superficial fungal infection that may occur anywhere and has nothing to do with worms. It usually involves dead tissues, such as the outer layer of skin, finger- or toenails, or hair. Several different fungi can cause these infections and it is difficult to distinguish among them, so they are considered as a group. On the feet, these infections are referred to as athlete's foot or ringworm of the feet; on the scalp or nails, often just as ringworm. Ringworm usually appears as small grayish scales with a raised border, the center of which may appear to be clearing up. Nails may be thickened and distorted and may eventually be destroyed if not treated. On the scalp ringworm is very common in children, especially in cities, and is highly infectious (spreads easily). To cure this infection, good hygiene is essential. Wash well and dry the area. Treat with the products listed below and keep after it until it is completely gone.

Fungal infections are some of the few ailments that over-the-counter agents can in fact cure, rather than just treat symptoms. In general, they are harder to treat and cure effectively than bacterial infections, and failures and recurrences are more common. Oral antifungal agents are not available over the counter, but topical treatment is best in nearly all cases because the drug is delivered directly to the site. Several of the best agents have been moved from prescription-only to over-the-counter status, making self-cures fairly easy. The key to curing the problem is to treat long enough. About 90% of infections are cured in four weeks. Specific agents for each of the categories are recommended, as well as alternatives.

Active Ingredients in Antifungals

Clotrimazole. Clotrimazole is an antibiotic (has both antibacterial and antifungal activity) used primarily for yeast and fungal infections. It is very effective for athlete's foot, jock itch, ringworm, diaper rash, candida (thrush), and vaginal yeast/fungal infections. Used since 1976, it is applied topically to the site. Adverse effects are rare, but some people may have burning or irritation at the site of application. **Pregnant women:** no evidence of risk. **Nursing mothers:** no evidence of risk. **Seniors:** no special problems. **Drug interactions:** topical use means low risk—none reported.

Miconazole. This second widely used and effective antifungal agent has been in use since the 1970s. It is equally useful for all of the indications noted for clotrimazole. Side effects are quite rare. **Pregnant women:** no evidence of risk. **Nursing mothers:** no evidence of risk. **Seniors:** no special problems. **Drug interactions:** topical use means low risk—none reported.

Tolnaftate. One of the early antifungals found to be effective topically, tolnaftate has been in use since 1965. It does not work as well as clotrimazole or miconazole, but is still effective for many cases of ringworm, athlete's foot, and jock itch. It does not seem to work well for fungal infections of the scalp, nails, palms of the hands, or soles of the feet. Adverse effects are rare and it does not generally cause irritation, but occasional stinging is reported. **Pregnant women:** no evidence of risk. **Nursing mothers:** no evidence of risk. **Seniors:** no special problems. **Drug interactions:** topical use means low risk—none reported.

Nystatin. Introduced in 1954, this antifungal was widely used to treat yeast infections. It is also not as effective as the newer agents, but continues to be available as an alternative in several products that are safe and effective for their intended use. It rarely causes side effects and can even be used by pregnant women to treat vaginal candidiasis. **Pregnant women:** no evidence of risk. **Nursing mothers:** no evidence of risk. **Seniors:** no special problems. **Drug interactions:** topical use means low risk—none reported.

Haloprogin. Haloprogin is a fungicidal agent (kills fungi) that is used in preparations for athlete's foot and other fungal infections of the skin. It is poorly absorbed, so it has few side effects except for occasional burning or irritation, especially on the feet. The cure rate is not as high as for clotrimazole or miconazole. Treatment should continue for three to four weeks. The relapse rate of fungal infections is also higher with this ingredient than for clotrimazole or miconazole. **Pregnant women:** no evidence of risk. **Nursing mothers:** no evidence of risk. **Seniors:** no special problems. **Drug interactions:** topical use means low risk—none reported.

Undecylenic acid. Undecylenic acid is a fungistatic agent (stops fungal growth). It is sometimes used in soap, but is not likely to be effective this way. The cure rate for this drug is lowest of the antifungal agents. It should be used for at least four weeks for best results. **Pregnant women:** no evidence of risk. **Nursing mothers:** no evidence of risk. **Seniors:** no special problems. **Drug interactions:** topical use means low risk—none reported.

Athlete's Foot, Diaper Rash, Jock Itch, Ringworm (Topical Use)

FIRST CHOICE *for seniors, adults, children*

Generic name: Clotrimazole *or* miconazole

Dose: Clotrimazole, 1% conc.; miconazole, 2 % conc.

Brand names: Lotrimin AF (cream and solution), Micatin (cream, powder, and spray)

Reasons: Both clotrimazole and miconazole are very effective and safe for topical use. They are equal in most respects.

Cautions: Side effects are very rare with these drugs and when used as directed should not cause any problems. They are nearly always effective in curing the infection.

Athlete's Foot, Diaper Rash, Jock Itch, Ringworm

SECOND CHOICE *for seniors, adults, children*

Generic name: Tolnaftate *or* nystatin

Dose: Tolnaftate, 1% conc.; nystatin, 1% conc.

Brand names: Aftate (gel, powder, or spray), Antifungal, Dr. Scholl's Athlete's Foot, Genaspor, NP-27 (aerosol, powder, cream), Tinactin, Ting (cream, powder, spray), Zeasorb-AF

Reasons: These second choice agents may be a little less expensive, but there is a bigger risk of not curing the infection. They are less effective and slower acting.

Cautions: These topically applied drugs have a very low incidence of adverse effects. Rarely, they may cause a local irritation, some redness, or a rash.

Athlete's Foot, Diaper Rash, Jock Itch, Ringworm

THIRD CHOICE *for seniors, adults, children*

Generic name: Haloprogin *or* undecylenic acid

Dose: Haloprogin, 5–20% conc.; undecylenic acid, 5–20% conc.

Brand names: Blis to Sol Liquid, Caldesene, Cruex Medicated (cream), Cruex Spray Powder, Decylenes, Desenex (cream, foam, liquid, ointment, powder), Merlenate, Quinsana Plus, Sal-Dex

Reasons: Haloprogin and undecylenic acid are the third choice of active ingredients because they have a lower level of success and rate of cure and are slower in eliminating fungal infections.

Cautions: Topical use and other properties limit the possible adverse effects of these drugs to local irritation, redness, and rash, none of which occurs with any regularity.

Hair Growth/Loss

The loss of hair or the failure to grow hair is a common problem associated with aging as well as numerous other conditions. It may also result from some types of drug therapy. Many millions of dollars are expended each year by those trying to stop hair loss or grow hair where it no longer grows. "Male pattern" baldness (loss of hair selectively from the top and/or front of the head) is very common. Although its cause is unknown, heredity appears to be the major factor. There is no cure, but several years ago, observers noticed that some patients taking a drug used in hypertension (high blood pressure) experienced hair growth as a side effect. Since that time, the drug has been marketed for promoting hair growth, and topical, prescription-only use has been advertised to the public. Unfortunately, only about one-third of those trying this treatment see any results, and that is usually limited to a very fine, thin growth of hair. The effect is slow to occur and is quite expensive. All over-the-counter preparations that claim to promote hair growth or prevent hair loss have been judged ineffective and are a waste of money.

Lice

Infections of the skin and hair by lice is a common problem where good hygiene is not practiced; but lice infestations can also be spread in a school environment or anywhere overcrowding, personal contact, or sharing of combs or other similar objects is common. Infestations are most frequent in September, October, and November. This infestation occurs routinely in about 3% of children nationwide each year normally, but up to 55% of 6-to-12-year-olds may be infected. It is more frequent in low-income neighborhood schools.

The lice themselves (small, flat, wingless insects with three pairs of legs) are hard to find, but their eggs can be easily discovered by careful examination of the hair and scalp. The eggs (nits) are tightly attached to the hair shafts and are difficult to remove. When the eggs hatch, the babies must have a blood meal within a few hours or they die. The bite is painless, but an allergic reaction usually develops. Itching is severe and frequent heavy scratching may break the skin and result in secondary bacterial infections of the resulting wounds. Other common sites of infection include the seams of clothing and in the pubic area, but also occasionally in the armpits, eyebrows, eyelashes, and beard. Cure is rapid and complete when instructions are followed, including using a fine comb to remove the eggs from the hair shafts after shampooing with the medicated shampoo.

Ingredients for Anti-Lice Therapy

Permethrin. Permethrin has rather recently been switched from prescription-only to over-the-counter availability. This anti-lice agent is very effective, resulting in a nearly 100% cure rate when used as directed. It is faster and more effective than products containing pyrethrin in effecting a cure, and has a lower incidence of side effects as well. **Pregnant women:** no evidence of risk. **Nursing mothers:** no evidence of risk. **Seniors:** no special problems. **Drug interactions:** topical use means low risk—none reported.

Pyrethrin. Moderately effective pediculocide (lice killer), which when combined with another ingredient is more effective. It is available in several preparations including gel, shampoo, and liquid products. **Pregnant women:** no evidence of risk. **Nursing mothers:** no evidence of risk. **Seniors:** no special problems. **Drug interactions:** topical use means low risk—none reported.

Head Lice (Topical Use)

FIRST CHOICE *for all ages*

Generic name: Permethrin

Dose: 1% conc.

Brand names: Nix

Reasons: Permethrin is the most effective, and very safe, ingredient for treating lice. When used as directed, it results in a rapid and complete cure in nearly every patient, every time it is used.

Cautions: None of concern.

Head Lice (Topical Use)

SECOND CHOICE *for all ages*

Generic name: Pyrethrin

Dose: 0.3% conc.

Brand names: (shampoo, gel, and foam) A-200 Pyrinate, Barc, Lice-Enz, Licetrol, Pronto, R & C, RID, Tisit, Triple X

Reasons: A less effective product than the first choice, pyrethrin offers an alternative in case of any dissatisfaction with the number one choice.

Cautions: None of concern.

Poison Ivy/Oak/Sumac

These plants are responsible for a large proportion of skin diseases. The first time you are exposed, you may see little or no response, but on subsequent exposure, the skin eruption is often very severe. Each of the plants contains related antigens which, unlike many other allergens, induces an allergic response in virtually everyone exposed to the plants. The resulting inflammation of the skin is very uncomfortable, and in severe cases can be debilitating.

The rash usually develops a day or two after exposure. A red, weeping rash covers only the area exposed, or areas that have been scratched or rubbed after touching the exposed area, spreading the oil-like sensitizing material. The rash feels hot, is swollen, and itches intensely. Many little blisters frequently form. It generally takes two or three weeks for the rash to heal completely. Prevention is nearly impossible, because the reaction starts within minutes after exposure. If you know you have contacted one of these plants, you must wash with soap within about ten minutes or it's too late. These rashes cannot be spread to others except within a short time after exposure, by transfer of the oil/resin through touch, or from contaminated clothing. Smoke from burning these plants can also get on the skin and induce the allergic reaction.

Effective Ingredients for Poison Ivy/Oak/Sumac

Anti-inflammatory: hydrocortisone. This drug is actually a hormone produced naturally by the body. It is used topically to relieve itch and irritation because it has potent anti-inflammatory effects. It is very effective for a wide variety of diseases and provides relief of several symptoms. Overuse may lead to permanent thinning of the skin as well as other more serious (but rare) adverse effects. **Pregnant women:** no evidence of risk. **Nursing mothers:** no evidence of risk. **Seniors:** no special problems, but to reduce possibility of skin thinning, prolonged use should be once daily and perhaps lower concentration products used if effective. **Drug interactions:** topical use means low risk.

Astringents: calamine or zinc oxide. These agents act on the surface to protect and soften diseased, damaged, or dead layers of skin. They are soothing and help to reduce itching and irritation. There are many related drugs and some distinctions among their effects can be made, but superiority overall is hard to establish. **Pregnant women:** no evidence of risk. **Nursing mothers:** no evidence of risk. **Seniors:** no special problems.

Local anesthetic: benzocaine. Introduced 85 years ago, benzocaine is one of the first and still one of the best local anesthetics. It is used in many diverse formulations for relief of surface pain and also to relieve itching. It is very poorly absorbed through the skin or mucous membranes, making it quite safe for use. It has few adverse effects, though occasionally a person may become allergic. **Pregnant women:** no evidence of risk. **Nursing mothers:** no evidence of risk. **Seniors:** no special problems. **Drug interactions:** topical use means low risk—none reported.

Local anesthetic: lidocaine. Lidocaine is a local anesthetic with a rapid onset of effect. It has more penetrating ability (through the skin and mucous membranes) and longer duration (about one hour) than benzocaine. It is widely available in different products for pain and itching. Used for over 40 years, it is also quite safe and effective. **Pregnant women:** no evidence of risk. **Nursing mothers:** no evidence of risk. **Seniors:** no special problems. **Drug interactions:** topical use means low risk—none reported.

Local anesthetic: dibucaine. Dibucaine is a very potent local anesthetic and quite long lasting in its effects. Due to these properties, it also has a higher incidence of undesirable side effects (allergy, headache, dizziness). It is most useful for prolonged relief and when the maximum anesthetic effect is desired. **Pregnant women:** no evidence of risk. **Nursing mothers:** no evidence of risk. **Seniors:** no special problems. **Drug interactions:** topical use means low risk—none reported.

Antihistamine: diphenhydramine. Diphenhydramine is one of the oldest and most common antihistamines. Its widespread, long-term use has proven it to be very safe. Due to a high incidence of characteristic side effects, it is also used as a sleeping aid, cough suppressant, and anti-nausea drug. **Pregnant women:** no evidence of risk. **Nursing mothers:** no evidence of risk. **Seniors:** no special problems by topical route. **Drug interactions:** topical use means low risk—none reported.

Poison Ivy/Oak/Sumac (Topical Use)

FIRST CHOICE *for seniors, adults, children*

Generic name: Hydrocortisone

Dose: 0.5–1% conc.

Creams: Anusol HC-1, Bactine, CaldeCORT, Cortaid, Cortizone-5, Dermacort, Dermolate, Dermtex HC, Foille-Cort, H2 Cort, Hydrocortisone, Hydro-Tex, Hytone, Lanacort, Pharmacort, Preparation HC, Racet SE, Rhulicort

Lotions: Cortaid, Delacort, Dermacort, Hydrocortisone, Rhulicort

Ointments: Cortaid, Cortizone-5,

Sprays: Cortaid

Reasons: Hydrocortisone is clearly the most effective topical treatment for skin rashes of many types, particularly allergic reactions. It may be used three times a day for a faster onset of effect, but after the first day or two, once a day is probably just as effective as more frequent use. For dry, scaly, eczema-type skin rashes, a greasy (ointment) formulation is best. For oozing or crusty lesions, the cream forms are superior.

Cautions: Excessive use of hydrocortisone preparations can lead to problems locally, or in extreme cases, even to general toxic effects, if too much is absorbed. Thinning of the skin (which can be permanent) is the most serious problem, and some increased susceptibility to infection (especially if the skin is broken) may result. When used as directed on the label, these products are some of the safest and most effective agents available for over-the-counter use to relieve the inflammation and irritation of skin rashes.

Poison Ivy/Oak/Sumac (Topical Use)

SECOND CHOICE *for seniors, adults, children*

Generic name: Diphenhydramine (antihistamine) *with* calamine or zinc oxide (astringent) *and* benzocaine (anesthetic)

Dose: See label

Brand names: Caladryl, Calmatum, Dalicote, Ivarest, Poison Ivy Spray, RhuliCream, RhuliSpray, Ziradryl

Reasons: Little information is available on this class of agents as far as whether any particular formulation is better than the others. The classes of drugs used are effective individually for the symptoms that are seen in poison ivy/oak/sumac reactions, and therefore they are presumed to be among the best combination agents for use in treating this skin rash. Antihistamines are more effective if taken by mouth, but are also included in many topically applied preparations and may provide some benefit.

Cautions: The topical use of antihistamines, astringents, and anesthetics is quite safe and adverse effects are rare. Occasionally an individual will become allergic to one or more of the ingredients, and the application will cause a rash or irritation to the skin. Other than this, there is little to be concerned about with these drugs and they may be quite helpful in treating the symptoms of rashes.

Psoriasis

Affecting about 3–5% of all age segments of the population, psoriasis is characterized by distinctive red patches of skin covered with silvery scales. An excessive buildup of skin cells occurs in certain areas, usually the scalp, elbows, and buttocks. The cause of this disease is unknown. Onset is usually gradual, and the disease has periods of quiescence and times when it flares up. It may also be seen, especially in children, when spots from chicken pox are healing. Sunlight appears to help this condition, and other treatments, as noted below, can be very effective as well.

Effective, Active Ingredients for Psoriasis

Coal tar and salicylic acid. Either one of these agents can be used alone, but they are more effective when combined. Together, they form a team that has some antifungal activity and the ability to remove dead skin. **Pregnant women:** no evidence of risk. **Nursing mothers:** no evidence of risk. **Seniors:** no special problems. **Drug interactions:** topical use means low risk—none reported.

Hydrocortisone. This drug is actually a hormone produced naturally by the body. Its potent anti-inflammatory effects make it ideal for topical relief of itching and irritation. It is used for a wide variety of diseases and provides relief of several symptoms. Overuse may lead to permanent thinning of the skin as well as other more serious (but rare) adverse effects. **Pregnant women:** no evidence of risk. **Nursing mothers:** no evidence of risk. **Seniors:** no special problems, but preferably use once per day for long-term use to reduce possibility of skin thinning. **Drug interactions:** topical use means low risk.

Psoriasis (Topical Use)

FIRST CHOICE *for seniors, adults, children*

Generic name: Hydrocortisone

Dose: 0.5–1% conc.

Creams: Anusol HC-1, Bactine, CaldeCORT, Cortaid, Cortizone-5, Dermacort, Dermolate, Dermtex HC, Foille-Cort, H2 Cort, Hydrocortisone, Hydro-Tex, Hytone, Lanacort, Pharmacort, Preparation HC, Racet SE, Rhulicort

Lotions: Cortaid, Delacort, Dermacort, Hydrocortisone, Rhulicort

Ointments: Cortaid, Cortizone-5

Reasons: Hydrocortisone is clearly the best topical treatment for skin rashes of many types, particularly allergic reactions. It may be used three times a day for a faster onset of effect, but after the first day or two, once a day is probably just as effective as more frequent use. For dry, scaly, eczema-type skin rashes, a greasy (ointment) formulation is best.

Cautions: The excessive use of hydrocortisone preparations can lead to problems locally or, in extreme cases, even to general toxic effects, if too much is absorbed. Thinning of the skin (which can be permanent) is the most serious problem, and some increased susceptibility to infection (especially if the skin is broken) may result. When used as directed, these products are some of the safest and most effective agents available for over-the-counter use.

Psoriasis (Topical Use)

SECOND CHOICE *for seniors, adults, children*

Generic name: Coal tar *or* salicylic acid *with* sulfur

Dose: Coal tar, 2% conc.; salicylic acid, 1–3 % conc.; sulfur, 2.5 % conc.

Brand names: Diasporal, Glover's Medicated Ointment, SLT Lotion, Tarlene, Vanseb

Reasons: This class of product is a combination agent, which is better than any of the single agents alone. It is generally well accepted by patients for reasons of smell, side effects, and the overall esthetics of use.

Cautions: None of special concern.

Scabies

A skin disease characterized by intense itching, scabies is caused by the itch mite (a very tiny animal that burrows into the skin). Particularly common under conditions of war or other poor sanitation, the mite infests the skin and lays eggs that cause the intense itching. It is easily transmitted, especially within a family. The itching is most intense at night and most commonly involves the genitals of men; spaces between the fingers, wrists, elbows, other skin folds; around the nipples of the breasts in women; along the belt line, and on the buttocks. In infants, the face may be involved. Scratching, and the resulting rash and irritation, may obscure the initial lesions made by the mite. A long hot bath, with vigorous cleansing and application of permethrin cream (see below) will rapidly and effectively cure the problem. This problem is often not recognized because the skin rash may resemble those caused by other factors.

Ingredient for Scabies

Permethrin. Permethrin has recently been switched from prescription-only to over-the-counter availability. This anti-lice/anti-scabies agent is very effective, resulting in a nearly 100% cure rate when used as directed. **Pregnant women:** no evidence of risk. **Nursing mothers:** no evidence of risk. **Seniors:** no special problems. **Drug interactions:** topical use means low risk—none reported.

Scabies

FIRST CHOICE

Generic name: Permethrin

Dose: 5% conc.

Brand names: Nix

Reasons: Permethrin is the best agent that is both safe and effective for killing mites.

Cautions: This topically applied therapy is very safe, and side effects, including itching, redness, or swelling of the area of application, rarely occurs when used as directed.

Seborrhea

For many years this skin disease was poorly understood. Now it seems very clear that it is similar to dandruff, both being caused by yeast infections of the skin (the scalp for dandruff and other areas for seborrhea). The newer antifungal drugs, also very effective for many yeast infections, have dramatically improved the treatment of this skin rash. There are a number of agents for treatment of this condition, which are described under "Dandruff and Seborrhea" on page 129. The choices for treatment of seborrhea differ somewhat from those for dandruff.

Seborrhea (Topical Use)

FIRST CHOICE *for seniors, adults, children*

Generic name: Selenium sulfide *or* zinc pyrithione

Dose: Selenium sulfide, 1% conc.; zinc pyrithione, 1–2% conc.

Brand names: Breck One, Selenium sulfide

Reasons: Very little toxicity or side effects occur with selenium sulfide and zinc pyrithione. They have antimicrobial activity, and gradual improvement is noted in most patients over several weeks of use.

Cautions: None of special concern.

Seborrhea (Topical Use)

SECOND CHOICE *for seniors, adults, children*

Generic name: Coal tar *or* salicylic acid *with* sulfur

Dose: Coal tar, 2% conc.; salicylic acid, 1–3% conc.; sulfur, 2.5 % conc.

Brand names: Diasporal, Glover's Medicated Ointment, SLT Lotion, Tarlene, Vanseb

Reasons: This group of products is a combination agent, which is better than any of the single agents. It is generally well accepted by patients for reasons of more pleasant smell, fewer side effects, and the overall better esthetics of use. They are less effective than the first choice products, but may be preferred nonetheless. The antifungal activity of coal tar is minimal, which is why the combination is recommended.

Cautions: None of special concern.

Skin Protectants

Barrier creams are frequently used to protect the skin from exposure to chemicals or to prevent poison ivy/oak/sumac contact allergic reactions. They are topically applied and form a film that protects the skin. This is very difficult to do without leaving the skin greasy or interfering with dexterity or touch sensitivity. Some creams are intended to be water repellant and are usually very greasy. Others are oil- or solvent-resistant, but then they come off in water. Whether or not such products are effective is still not clear. Adequate testing has not been performed. At this point, the specialized products have not been proven any better than petrolatum or anhydrous lanolin.

Active Ingredients for Protecting the Skin

Petrolatum. Petrolatum is the best skin softener/moisturizer/protectant (emollient) for a variety of diseases and symptoms. This ointment (water in oil) product serves to protect and shield the skin from irritating substances by taking up water and forming an occlusive barrier to prevent the loss of water. An alternative is animal fat-derived *lanolin* but, because many people are or can become allergic to this wool fat, it is not highly recommended. Other alternatives include *mineral oil* and various *vegetable oils* (like *cocoa butter*), but no clear advantages or additional arguments for their use over petrolatum have been proven. **Pregnant women:** no evidence of risk. **Nursing mothers:** no evidence of risk. **Seniors:** no special problems. For more information, see "Diaper Rash," on page 132.

Sunburn

Nearly everyone experiences sunburn at one time or another. The best treatment is prevention: limiting your exposure to the sun by staying in the shade, covering the skin, or applying sunscreens. When these measures fail, there are a number of effective actions to reduce the pain and foster rapid healing. None of the drugs for sunburn, available over the counter or by prescription, have been shown to cure the damage already inflicted by overexposure to the sun, but the following measures are best. As soon as possible, take an oral analgesic/anti-inflammatory agent to reduce pain, erythema (redness), and edema (swelling) (see Chapter 2, page 21). Cold water or ice compresses can be applied directly as soon as pain is noted to reduce the burning effect. Topical steroid creams (hydrocortisone) also seem to reduce redness if used very early (see page 115). To supplement the oral analgesic, topical anesthetics (see Chapter 3, page 38) can be applied, and lotions may be used to reduce the drying of the skin (see page 136). Sunburn may produce fever, dehydration, and even shock. Drink plenty of liquids to prevent dehydration. The topical local anesthetics of preference are benzocaine, lidocaine, and dibucaine. See "Burns," page 124, for products and dosages.

Warts

The occurrence of these unsightly growths on the skin is a common (estimated at 7–10% of the population) dermatological affliction, affecting particularly the young and peaking in the 12-16-year-old age range. Warts are caused by a large number of related viruses, and can be difficult to cure. To be successful, the treatment must be intense and consistent, using the best available products. If over-the-counter drug measures are ineffective, there are several surgical methods that are more expensive and painful, but which will effect cures in the majority of even difficult cases. Because some of the over-the-counter agents do not work, many people do not realize that a self-cure can be effected.

Although the exact mode of spread is unknown, it is clear that the virus enters the skin after contact with an infected person or surface, and that an incubation period of one to eight months is required before the warts become noticeable. Treatment can not only cure the problem, it also reduces the spread of the lesions, so it should be initiated as soon as possible. Common warts can occur anywhere on the skin, and can usually be treated effectively. Plantar warts, which afflict the bottom of the feet, may take a very concerted and conscientious effort over a longer period of time to effect a cure. Plantar warts are extremely common and can be painful and debilitating, since instead of growing on the surface of the skin, they grow into the foot and usually on pressure areas of close contact between bones in the foot and the ground. The knowledge about these viral infections is limited and many folklore methods are touted as effective. The natural history of warts is that in most cases they will go away on their own within two years. Below is a summary of the preferred treatments.

Active Ingredient for Warts

Salicylic acid. This agent is a derivative of aspirin, which has pronounced properties to remove a layer(s) of skin cells. It is used topically to treat acne, and also in higher concentrations for wart and corn and callus removal and similar uses. Treatment should be continued over several weeks. For best results, soak the wart site for five minutes in warm water, and then remove as much of the wart (an emery board works well) as possible without causing bleeding. Apply the salicylic acid and cover the site with waterproof tape to keep the site moist. **Pregnant women:** no evidence of risk. **Nursing mothers:** no evidence of risk. **Seniors:** no special problems. **Drug interactions:** topical use means very low risk—none reported.

Warts (Topical Use)

FIRST CHOICE *for seniors, adults, children*

Generic name: Salicylic acid

Dose: 26–40% conc.

Brand names: Occlusal-HP

Reasons: This preparation of salicylic acid is more irritating than those listed below, but the cure rate is higher and faster.

Cautions: This drug can be irritating, and depending on the tolerance of the individual, may have to be applied for a few hours at a time on successive days rather than used continuously.

Warts (Topical Use)

SECOND CHOICE *for seniors, adults, children*

Generic name: Salicylic acid

Dose: 17% conc.

Brand names: Compound W Wart Remover, Duofilm, Dr. Scholl's Wart Remover Kit, Occlusal, Off Ezy Wart Removal Kit, Trans-Ver-Sal, Wart-Off

Reasons: These products contain a lower concentration of the active, effective ingredient and will therefore require a longer treatment period, or may not be completely effective in removing the wart(s). The secret to curing warts is a concerted effort over several weeks to get rid of the virus.

Cautions: These products are very safe for use, and the only problem is likely to be some irritation of the normal skin around the wart, if the products are not confined to the wart.

Wounds and Injuries

The skin does a very good job of protecting itself from infections. It provides a protective layer that keeps bacteria, fungi, yeast, and viruses from producing an infection most of the time. Occasionally, hair follicles or sweat glands can become infected, resulting in *boils* or *carbuncles*. Damage to the skin can result in superficial fungal or bacterial infections, or cuts and scrapes may allow the establishment of skin infections, which can then spread into the blood in severe cases. Only the most minor skin infections should be self-treated. Most of the effort in this area is directed at preventing the development of infections. When the skin is damaged, it is important to wash the wound well with soap and water. Antiseptics (which kill bacteria) then may be applied to reduce the possibility of infection. Most are not very effective or have a very limited duration.

Antibiotic creams may also be used. Although usually not necessary, they can provide some benefit, may hasten healing, and probably provide some peace of mind. Studies to evaluate the usefulness of prophylactic antibiotic use, or even the use of antiseptics, have not provided clear-cut answers. The benefit is apparently small, but the use of such agents may reduce infections, particularly if the injury occurred outdoors, was due to broken glass, or resulted in exposure to many germs (bacteria). Proper cleaning, or even soaking in warm salt water, seems to be as effective as antibiotic or antiseptic treatment. The wound should be kept covered and moist, while allowing air access. It should also be insulated from hot or cold extremes and protected from secondary infection using bandages. Complete healing requires about two weeks.

Active Ingredients for Wounds and Injuries

Polymyxin B. A bactericidal agent (kills bacteria) that is active on the surface to prevent or cure infections. Polymixin B is not absorbed, thereby reducing the possibility of side effects, but also limiting its effect to the surface. Resistance of bacteria to this drug is rare, making it very useful and effective in that regard. **Pregnant women:** no evidence of risk. **Nursing mothers:** no evidence of risk. **Seniors:** no special problems. **Drug interactions:** topical use means very low risk—none reported.

Bacitracin. Used since 1948, bacitracin is another antibiotic that acts by a different mechanism and on a different group of bacteria than the Polymyxin B described above. It is also for topical use and has a very low incidence of side effects (rarely an allergic reaction may develop). It is used in combination with other agents to have a very broad effect. **Pregnant women:** no evidence of risk. **Nursing mothers:** no evidence of risk. **Seniors:** no special problems. **Drug interactions:** topical use means very low risk—none reported.

Neomycin sulfate. Another long-used agent, this is a broad spectrum antibiotic (meaning it is effective against many different bacteria). It is also very effective and safe for topical use, although of all the agents in this group, it probably has the most likelihood of inducing an allergic reaction in the skin. **Pregnant women:** no evidence of risk. **Nursing mothers:** no evidence of risk. **Seniors:** no special problems. **Drug interactions:** topical use means very low risk—none reported.

Tetracycline. A broad spectrum bacteriostatic agent, tetracycline is effective against a wide variety of bacteria (often used for acne). Although it is not used as frequently as the combination of the other agents described above, it is a good alternative if there should be any irritation or allergy to the triple combination (first choice). **Pregnant women:** no evidence of risk. **Nursing mothers:** no evidence of risk. **Seniors:** no special problems. **Drug interactions:** topical use means very low risk—none reported.

Wounds, Cuts, Scrapes (Topical Antibiotics)

FIRST CHOICE *for seniors, adults, children*

Generic name: Polymyxin B *and* bacitracin *and* neomycin sulfate

Dose: See label

Brand names: Bactine First Aid Antibiotic, Lanabiotic Ointment, Medi-Quik, Mycitracin, N.B.P., Neomixin, Neosporin, Neo-Thrycex, Septa, Trimycin, Triple Antibiotic

Reasons: The combination of these three antibiotics gives the broadest possible coverage of anti-infective potential. Each of the three has a different spectrum of germs that it kills, and combined, their ability to effect a cure of surface infections is maximized.

Cautions: As with nearly all topically applied drugs, the main potential side effect is developing an allergic reaction to the drug(s). This problem is fairly minor, and the number of people that become allergic is small but must be considered, especially if the infection is not cured quickly or the site remains or becomes irritated after a few days of use.

Wounds, Cuts, Scrapes (Topical Antibiotics)

SECOND CHOICE *for seniors, adults, children*

Generic name: Tetracycline *or* single / double mix of first choice triple combination (described above)

Dose: See label

Brand names: Acromycin, Aureomycin, Baciguent, Bacitracin, Myciguent, Neomycin, Neosporin Cream, Polysporin (ointment and powder), Terramycin

Reasons: The single agent, or combination of two, does not have as broad a spectrum of antibiotic activity as the first choice; but these products are a good alternative if for some reason the first choice is not effective, or you are allergic to one of the three antibiotics used in the first choice products.

Cautions: There are few adverse effects from topical use of these agents. The occasional development of an allergic reaction is about the only side effect to watch for. These reactions are not serious and by discontinuing use of the drug, the rash or irritation will go away.

Yeast Infections

Yeast infections of the skin and mucous membranes by candida can lead to very inflamed and uncomfortable rashes. These infections tend to occur on the skin in the groin area, under the arms, in folds of skin under the breasts, between the toes, around the anus, and in the diaper area of infants. Mucous membranes, including the mouth (thrush) and vagina (see Chapter 9, page 190 for treatment) are also susceptible areas. Yeast generally produces a bright red, painful lesion, characterized by burning rather than itching. A "moth-eaten" appearance to skin is often noted. Hot, humid conditions and occlusive clothing or shoes often precipitate these infections. Affected areas should be treated topically with the agents described and the affected area should be exposed to the air. Wear only loose cotton garments if possible. Eating yogurt may also help to reestablish the normal flora for infections of the anal, vaginal, and diaper areas.

Active Ingredients for Yeast Infections

Clotrimazole. This antibiotic (has both antibacterial and antifungal activity) is used primarily for yeast and fungal infections. It is very effective for athlete's foot, jock itch, ringworm, diaper rash, candida (thrush), and vaginal yeast/fungal infections. Used since 1976, it is applied topically to the site. Adverse effects are rare, but some people may have burning or irritation at the site of application. **Pregnant women:** no evidence of risk. **Nursing mothers:** no evidence of risk. **Seniors:** no special problems. **Drug interactions:** topical use means very low risk—none reported.

Miconazole. This widely used and effective antifungal agent has been in use since the 1970s. It is also useful for all of the indications noted for clotrimazole, and the two drugs really cannot be distinguished from one another in the therapy of these indications. Side effects are quite rare. **Pregnant women:** no evidence of risk. **Nursing mothers:** no evidence of risk. **Seniors:** no special problems. **Drug interactions:** topical use means very low risk—none reported.

Yeast Infections (Topical Use)

FIRST CHOICE *for seniors, adults, children*

Generic name: Clotrimazole *or* miconazole

Dose: Clotrimazole, 1% conc.; miconazole, 2% conc.

Brand names: Lotrimin AF (cream and solution), Micatin (cream, powder, and spray)

Reasons: Both clotrimazole and miconazole are very effective and safe for topical use. They are equal in most respects.

Cautions: Side effects are very rare with these drugs, and when used as directed should not cause any problems, but are nearly always effective in curing the infection.

Oral Products for Treatment of Skin Problems

Although in most cases the most efficient and effective treatment of skin problems is by direct application of medicine to the skin, some skin problems are better handled by oral treatment. This is true for allergic reactions when relief of itching is the desired effect or when sunburn is the problem and pain relief is the goal. The topical agents do not penetrate very far into the skin and are less effective than oral administration of the relatively specific treatments provided by antihistamine and analgestic over-the-counter drugs. Specific products and optimal treatments are described below.

Allergy/Skin Rash (Oral Use)

FIRST CHOICE *for seniors, adults, children*

Generic name: Chlorpheniramine *or* brompheniramine

Dose: Chlorpheniramine, 2–4 mg (8–12 mg long acting); brompheniramine, 2–12 mg

Tablets: Aller-Chlor, Chlor-Trimeton (long acting and maximum strength), Dimetane, Pfeiffer's Allergy, Teldrin

Liquids: Aller-Chlor, Chlor-Trimeton, Dimetane,

Reasons: For relief of hives or allergic skin reactions, the best treatment is the single-agent product, rather than the combination drugs. An antihistamine is the most effective, supplemented by topical steroid application (see page 69) if needed to help relieve the itching. These are the best of the antihistamines.

Cautions: All of the antihistamines that are available over the counter have sedation or drowsiness as a potential side effect. The least sedating of these is chlorpheniramine, the one recommended here. It also has a good duration of effect so that it doesn't have to be taken in as large a dose or as often as many others.

Allergy/Skin Rash (Oral Use)

SECOND CHOICE *for seniors, adults, children*

Generic names: Diphenhydramine *or* triprolidine

Dose: Diphenhydramine, 25–50 mg; triprolidine, 1.25–2.5 mg

Tablets: Actidil, Aller-Max, Banophen, Benadryl, Genahist, Nidryl

Liquids: Actidil, Genahist, Nidryl, Phendry

Reasons: The products listed here are also plain antihistamines. They have ingredients that are somewhat more sedating than the first choice listed above. Diphenhydramine has a particularly long history of use by millions of people and is considered to be very safe and effective.

Cautions: These agents have a significant potential to induce drowsiness or decrease alertness. Follow the cautions against operating machinery or doing tasks requiring a high level of alertness.

Sunburn (Oral Use)

FIRST CHOICE *for seniors, adults, children*

Generic name: Ibuprofen

Dose: 200–400 mg/dose

Maximum: 2,400 mg/day

Brand names: Addaprin, Advil, Genpril, Haltran, Medipren, Motrin IB, Nuprin, Ultraprin, Valprin

Reasons: Although ibuprofen is somewhat more expensive than aspirin or acetaminophen, it is the most effective analgesic and is safer to use than aspirin. It provides pain relief and fever reduction and counters inflammation. Take it with meals to prevent stomach upset, which may occur in some people.

Cautions: Ibuprofen may cause stomach upset (nausea or vomiting) and rarely can cause ulcers (much less than aspirin). Diarrhea or constipation may occur in some people. It is not recommended for pregnant or breast-feeding women. Patients with kidney disease should consult a physician before using these products. Ibuprofen may interact with antihypertensive (blood pressure) drugs, diuretics (water pills), alcohol, antacids, and anticoagulants (blood thinners). Consult your physician if you take these medications. **Pregnant women:** not usually recommended. **Nursing mothers:** no evidence of risk to infant. **Seniors:** reduced dose may be desirable.

Sunburn (Oral Use)

SECOND CHOICE *for seniors, adults, children*

Generic name: Aspirin

Dose: 325–850 mg/dose

Brand names: Anacin, Bayer Aspirin, Ecotrin, Empirin, Norwich Aspirin, St. Joseph Aspirin, many others

Reasons: Aspirin is the standard for pain relief and fever reduction. It is also very inexpensive and is anti-inflammatory. Aspirin has more stomach upset (nausea and vomiting) associated with its use, and a higher potential for causing ulcers than ibuprofen. It is therefore less desirable overall. Risks of overdose are also more significant with aspirin.

Cautions: Thousands of cases of aspirin overdose occur each year because people do not respect this drug for what it really is, a potent, effective drug with significant toxicity. Heavy use induces significant damage to the stomach lining (ulcers) and may also result in nutrient depletion (especially iron). It interacts with antidiabetic drugs and anticoagulants (blood thinners). **Pregnant women:** not usually recommended. **Nursing mothers:** aspirin passes into the milk. **Seniors:** no special problems.

7

Eye Care

Although there are a number of conditions that can cause problems with the eyes, the most common problem is tired, red, irritated eyes from being awake too long or doing work that strains the eyes. Agents to remove the redness can provide temporary relief. The "dry eye" problem is also common, often as a result of wearing contact lenses. Significantly, many people who wear contacts or who have dry eye use ophthalmic preparations that contain preservatives and the preservatives are often the cause of the problem. The preservative benzalkonium chloride (very commonly used) can cause tear problems and irritate the eye. This chapter describes the agents and their optimal use for each of the problems mentioned.

Allergy

Itching is another common symptom for eyes, and this symptom suggests that an allergic disease is the culprit. If an allergic reaction is responsible for irritating your eyes and causing them to be red, watery, or itchy, the topical options are very limited. For redness, the products described later in this chapter can be used. However, for allergic reactions the best choice is an antihistamine. No over-the-counter topical antihistamines are available, and it is not even clear if they are, in fact, effective. You can get some relief by using oral antihistamines (see Chapter 4, page 69).

Dry Eyes

Dryness of the eye is a common, irritating problem, with many causes. Tears have several functions and are constantly produced and renewed by the blinking action to protect, lubricate, and cleanse the eyes. A variety of eye defects all produce similar symptoms. Itching is usually a symptom due to allergic reactions, but dry eye may be due to numerous diverse causes. The treatment is best directed at the source of the problem if possible, but often artificial tears are the standby treatment. They serve as artificial lubricants rather than real replacements for tears. They must be used rather frequently to be effective, and because most contain preservatives, there are frequent problems associated with their use. For best results, unpreserved tears (at least at night) should be used. Ointments are even better than solutions because they provide more lubrication and moisture-holding capacity. The safest, most commonly used, and effective agents are described below.

Active Ingredients for Dry Eyes

Carboxymethylcellulose (CMC). CMC is a water-holding material that is not absorbed and is used for various indications. It is used in diet aids to add bulk to the stomach (it swells with water) as well as in the eye as an ingredient for artificial tears to relieve dryness by holding moisture. **Pregnant women:** no evidence of risk. **Nursing mothers:** no evidence of risk. **Seniors:** no special problems.

Polyvinyl alcohol (PVA). Another of the water-holding materials that is not absorbed, PVA acts locally to increase and hold moisture in the eye and to relieve the dry eye syndrome. **Pregnant women:** no evidence of risk. **Nursing mothers:** no evidence of risk. **Seniors:** no special problems.

Dry Eyes (Drops Without Preservatives)

FIRST CHOICE *for seniors, adults, children*

Generic name: Carboxymethylcellulose *or* polyvinyl alcohol

Dose: Carboxymethylcellulose, 1% solution; polyvinyl alcohol, 1.4 % solution

Brand names: Celluvisc, Murocel, Refresh

Reasons: The purpose of these agents is to relieve the dry, irritated feeling in the eyes. Many of the available products have been found to actually increase the discomfort. This is due to the preservatives that are used to keep the solutions sterile (they irritate the eyes directly, or may induce allergic reactions). For this reason, nonpreserved solutions appear to be the best treatment (see cautions below).

Cautions: Because these solutions do not have preservatives (chemicals added to prevent bacteria or other germs from growing in the solution), they can become contaminated just by being opened or more likely by being touched to the eyes or skin. Before use, examine the solution carefully to be sure that it is not cloudy and does not have any particles floating around in it. The solution should be completely clear and colorless, or it should not be used.

Dry Eyes (Drops with Mild Preservatives)

SECOND CHOICE *for seniors, adults, children*

Generic name: Polyvinyl alcohol *or* methylcellulose *or* other cellulose *and* edetate sodium *or* chlorobutanol (mild preservatives)

Dose: Polyvinyl alcohol, 1.4% solution *or* methylcellulose, 0.5% solution; edetate sodium, less than 0.15% *or* chlorobutanol, less than 0.55%

Brand names: Artificial Tears Solution, Lacril, Liquifilm Tears, TearGard, Tears Naturale II, Tears Plus

Reasons: As stated under the descriptions of the first choice products, preservatives are frequently a major contributor to the dry eye problem by causing more irritation. However, since preservatives keep the solutions sterile, especially when used over a longer period of time—they are necessary. These products were selected as the second choice agents because the preservatives that are used are mild and usually won't cause problems.

Cautions: The only concern here is the possibility that the preservatives used can irritate the eyes. If relief is not obtained after following the label directions, consider changing to a preparation without preservatives.

Dry Eyes (Drops with Preservatives)

THIRD CHOICE *for seniors, adults, children*

Generic name: Polyvinyl alcohol *or* methylcellulose *and* thimerosal *or* benzalkonium chloride (preser- vatives)

Dose: Same as second choice doses

Brand names: Adsorbotear, Akwa Tears, Hypotears, I-Liqui Tears, Isopto Alkaline, Just Tears, Liquifilm Forte, Milroy Artificial Tears, Moisture Drops, Murine, Muro Tears, Tearisol, Tears Naturale, Tears Renewed, Ultra Tears

Reasons: These artificial tear formulations are effective, but may cause irritation to the eyes because of the preservatives used to keep them sterile. If you notice problems or little or no relief, resort to the second or first choices to see if things improve.

Caution: These products contain the highest level of preservatives and those preservatives most likely to cause irritation of the eye. If relief is not obtained, switch to products without preservatives.

Eye Infections

There are no over-the-counter agents for treatment of eye infections. You must see your physician or ophthalmologist for a prescription topical antibiotic. Although most eyedrops contain antiseptics, they are in very low concentration. They are used as preservatives to keep germs from growing in the solution, and they are therefore not useful for treating eye infections.

Red, Irritated Eyes

The eyes are our window to the world, and are often taken as a reflection of our inner self. We tend to overwork our eyes and frequently abuse them with poor lighting, and inadequate rest. When they tire, or are exposed to irritating substances in our environment, they respond by getting red and causing discomfort. The redness is caused by dilation (enlargement) of blood vessels, a condition which can be readily reversed with several vasoconstrictive agents (blood-vessel shrinking drugs) available over the counter in many different products. This following section outlines the most common ingredients in this class that are safe and effective, and recommends products containing these ingredients.

Active Ingredients for Red, Irritated Eyes

Naphazoline. A long-acting topically applied decongestant particularly well suited for use in the eyes, naphazoline constricts blood vessels to take out the redness. In use for 50 years, it is very effective and safe for use, but does not help itching. **Pregnant women:** no evidence of risk by topical use, but avoid oral route or excessive use. **Nursing mothers:** no evidence of risk, but oral doses result in drug passing into milk. **Seniors:** no special problems topically; reduce oral dose. **Drug interactions:** topical use means very low risk—none reported.

Tetrahydrozoline. Tetrahydrozoline is very similar to naphazoline in its effectiveness, duration, and safety. Occasionally it may cause dilation of the pupils leading to blurred vision and sensitivity to light. This is more frequent in people with light-colored eyes. **Pregnant women:** no evidence of risk by topical use, but avoid excessive use. **Nursing mothers:** no evidence of risk, but drug can pass into the milk. **Seniors:** no special problems for topical use. **Drug interactions:** topical use means very low risk—none reported.

   Oxymetazoline. Another decongestant for topical use, oxymetazoline also acts by constricting (shrinking) the blood vessels in the eye. It has a longer-lasting effect, so two doses per day are sufficient. Oxymetazoline may be irritating if used frequently or for too long. **Pregnant women:** no evidence of risk by topical use, but avoid oral route or excessive use. **Nursing mothers:** no evidence of risk, but drug can pass into the milk. **Seniors:** no special problems for topical use. **Drug interactions:** topical use means very low risk—none reported.

   Phenylephrine. Phenylephrine is a common decongestant for relief of nasal and sinus congestion. It is used both orally and topically. It has more potential for side effects on heart rate and blood pressure (increases both) and on the nervous system (anxiety, tremor, insomnia) than the other two agents listed above, but this is very rare when it is used topically. Its shorter duration of effect means it must be used more frequently. **Pregnant women:** no evidence of risk by topical use, but avoid oral route or excessive use. **Nursing mothers:** no evidence of risk, but oral doses result in drug passing into milk. **Seniors:** no special problems for topical use; reduce oral dose. **Drug interactions:** topical use means very low risk—none reported.

Red, Irritated Eyes (Drops Without Preservatives)

FIRST CHOICE *for seniors, adults, children*

   Generic name: Naphazoline hydrochloride *or* oxymetazoline hydrochloride *or* phenylephrine *or* tetrahydrozoline

   Dose: Naphazoline hydrochloride, 0.012%; oxymetazoline hydrochloride, 0.025%; phenylephrine, 0.05%; tetrahydrozoline, 0.05%

   Brand names: Allerest Eye Drops, Eye-Zine, Occu-Phrin, Optised, Relief, Tetrahydrozoline hydrochloride

   Reasons: Preservatives frequently irritate the eyes and make the situation worse, so even for occasional use, the nonpreserved preparations are preferred. Because this leaves the solution vulnerable for contamination by germs, it must be checked before use (see Cautions).

Cautions: Due to the absence of preservatives in these products, they must be checked before use to be sure that they remain sterile. The solutions must be absolutely clear and colorless, with nothing floating around in them. If you notice any of these conditions, discard the drops and purchase a new bottle.

Red, Irritated Eyes (Drops with Low Amount of Preservatives)

SECOND CHOICE *for seniors, adults, children*

Generic name: Naphazoline hydrochloride *or* oxymetazoline hydrochloride *or* phenylephrine *or* tetrahydrozoline

Dose: Naphazoline hydrochloride, 0.012%; oxymetazoline hydrochloride, 0.025%; phenylephrine, 0.12%; tetrahydrozoline, 0.05%

Brand names: AK-Nefrin, Clear Eyes, Comfort Eye Drops, Degest 2, Isopto-Frin, OcuClear, Optigene III, Phenylzin, Prefrin Liquifilm, Soothe, VasoClear, Visine

Reasons: As stated under the first choice, preservatives are frequently a major contributor to the dry eye problem by causing more irritation. Since preservatives are important to keep the solutions sterile—especially when used over a long period of time—they are necessary. These products are selected as the second choice because the preservatives used are mild and usually won't cause problems.

Cautions: The only concern here is to be aware of the possibility that the preservatives can irritate the eyes. If relief is not obtained after following the label directions, consider changing to a preparation without preservatives.

8

Sleep Disorders

No single activity takes as much of our time as sleep; nor are many things as important for our well-being as getting an adequate amount of good quality sleep. We can postpone sleep for some time, albeit with some decrease in our performance. More often the problem associated with sleep is insomnia, when sleep just won't come or is not restful. Sleep is very difficult to regulate, and when disturbed or interrupted, that deficiency can cause many problems. The over-the-counter agents described and discussed here can help to some extent for acute problems, but often a longer term solution for a persistent problem will be needed. Also included in this chapter is a short discussion of alcohol, which is widely used in many drugs to make the ingredients dissolve. The only over-the-counter stimulant, *caffeine*, is discussed, and its appropriate use for several different indications is covered. Caffeine can be used to increase alertness, overcome drowsiness, and for other uses, including enhancing the pain relieving effects of oral analgesics.

Alcohol

Used since the dawn of history for both medicinal and recreational (social) purposes, alcohol was held for many years to be a remedy for practically all diseases—a magic elixir. It is now clear that the therapeutic value is very limited, and its perceived social value predominates. It has several local effects, including cooling the skin by evaporation (for use in fever reduction), and it can kill bacteria, also by topical application. By far the most pronounced effects of alcohol, taken internally, are on the central nervous system (brain). Many people view alcohol as a stimulant, but in fact, it is a depressant. The confusion comes from the initial depression of normal control systems that facilitate lowering of inhibitions and unrestrained activity in certain areas of the brain. Thought and motor functions become disrupted and self-restraint is reduced. Mood swings and emotional reactions are altered and exaggerated. Chronic use results in severe damage and the irreversible loss of organ function, particularly of the liver. It also often affects the brain.

Alcohol is used in many liquid medications to dissolve drugs that do not dissolve in water. It is also used for the same reason in many topically applied products. The dose obtained from these preparations is usually low, unless large and frequent doses of the medication are taken. Many of the cold and flu combination drugs, cough syrups, and similar remedies are 25–50% alcohol. The depressant effect of alcohol can combine with similar effects of antihistamines in these drugs to help induce drowsiness, which may be desirable. However, another effect of alcohol, that of disrupting the quality of sleep, makes this use of alcohol for promoting rest and recovery from illness of questionable overall value.

Alcohol is also frequently used to obtain relief from anxiety or stress. Whether or not this effect is significant and useful is hotly debated. In large enough doses, alcohol clearly alters the perception of anxiety and stress, probably in a manner similar to the effects seen on the perception of pain and fatigue. In all these cases a certain detachment from the reality of the situation occurs, and sensitivity to the unpleasant symptom is reduced as a consequence of the central nervous system depression.

Sleep Aids

Lack of sleep can sabotage your physical and mental performance. Clumsiness at simple tasks, loss of dexterity, and serious problems with higher mental abilities (the first thing to go is creativity) are common consequences of sleep deprivation. Not being able to fall asleep quickly and not getting a good night's rest are frequent complaints that affect us all at one time or another. After the age of 45, up to 33% of the population claims difficulty in falling or remaining asleep. It is usually not a big problem, and is often caused by unusual stress or excitement much of the time. It will usually correct itself. If treatment is necessary, there is only one over-the-counter agent that is accepted as safe and has been shown to be effective in controlled human testing. It is an antihistamine that has been used for many years and has a well-established track record to induce drowsiness. Both the speed of falling asleep and a reduction in the number of awakenings during the night are noted when diphenhydramine is taken as directed. In addition to taking this drowsiness-inducing drug, other things you can do to help fall asleep include: drink a soothing beverage (like milk), take a warm bath (not hot or cold), count sheep (yes, it really does work), close your eyes and think of a relaxing fantasy, or start at your toes and tense and relax each muscle group of your body. Alcohol may help you fall asleep, but the ensuing sleep will be fragmented and unsatisfying, so this is not a recommended alternative.

Active Ingredient in Sleep Aids

Diphenhydramine. Diphenhydramine is one of the oldest and most common antihistamines. Due to widespread and long-time use, it is recognized as very safe. Because of a high incidence of characteristic side effects, diphenhydramine is also used as a cough suppressant and anti-nausea drug. **Pregnant women:** no evidence of risk. **Nursing mothers:** no evidence of risk to infant, but passes into breast milk. **Seniors:** reduced dose may be desirable or increased side effects may occur. **Drug interactions:** alcohol and sedatives—increased sedation; MAOI (monoamine oxidase inhibitor) drugs (certain antidepressants)—risk of hypertension (high blood pressure).

Sleep Aids

FIRST CHOICE *for seniors, adults, children*

Generic name: Diphenhydramine

Dose: 50 mg

Brand names: Compoz, Dormarex 2, Nervine Nighttime Sleep-Aid, Nytol, Sleep-Eze 3, Sleepinal, Sominex 2, Twilite Caplets

Reasons: Diphenhydramine is an antihistamine (used for allergies) with a side effect of inducing drowsiness. This property is sufficiently useful to make this product the only safe and effective over-the-counter drug to help induce sleep.

Cautions: Other side effects of antihistamines, other than the desired drowsiness, include dry mouth, dizziness, and blurred vision.

Sleep Aids (with Pain Relief)

FIRST CHOICE *for seniors, adults*

Generic name: Diphenhydramine *and* ibuprofen

Dose: Diphenhydramine, 50 mg; ibuprofen, see Chapter 2, page 21

Reasons: Take ibuprofen for the pain (see page 21) and diphenhydramine to induce drowsiness.

Cautions: The desired effect of drowsiness induced by this treatment is the major side effect to be aware of. Additionally, dry mouth, dizziness, and (rarely) blurred vision may occur if the dose is pushed. For the ibuprofen, stomach upset is the most frequent problem, but can be avoided by taking the drug with food. See detailed discussion of each drug for more information.

Sleep Aids (with Pain Relief)

SECOND CHOICE *for seniors, adults*

Generic name: Diphenhydramine *and* acetaminophen *or* aspirin

Dose: Diphenhydramine, 50 mg; acetaminophen *or* aspirin, see Chapter 2, page 31

Brand names: Arthritis Foundation Nighttime, Bayer Select Night Time Pain, Bufferin AF Nite Time, Excedrin PM, Quiet World Tablets, Sominex Pain Relief Formula, Tega S-A Tablets, Tylenol PM, Tylenol Cold Night Time, Unisom Dual Relief

Reasons: None of these products contains the first choice analgesic (ibuprofen). They do contain an acceptable alternative and the first (only) choice of sleep aids (diphenhydramine).

Cautions: The cautions are those applicable to the agents used in these products. Aspirin overdose can result from simultaneous use of multiple products containing aspirin, causing stomach irritation and possible ulcers. Acetaminophen is quite safe, but serious toxicity is possible with an overdose. See the cautions listed for diphenhydramine earlier in this section.

Stimulants

The only safe and effective over-the-counter agent in this category, caffeine, is used so heavily by so many people that it loses its potential effectiveness from overuse. It must be used constantly to maintain a "normal" state of alertness. It is found in coffee, many soft drinks, many pain relievers, and numerous other combination drugs for colds, aches and pains, diet aids, decongestants, menstrual relief products, and so on. This drug's ability to affect mood, alertness, and the ability to perform certain tasks has been recognized for many years. Virtually all cultures have developed customs and methods to acquire this drug on a routine basis.

Stimulant Ingredient

Caffeine. Caffeine is a naturally occurring drug found in several plants and used very widely for its stimulatory effects. Most cultures have traditional beverages containing caffeine, which are heavily used. It stimulates the central nervous system and usually produces decreased drowsiness, less fatigue, and a more rapid and clear flow of thought. Enhancing effects on concentration, reflex time, and other tasks are also noted. Additional effects of this drug include stimulation of water loss by effects on the kidney, stimulation of the heart muscle, and relaxation of smooth muscle. Caffeine has also been shown to enhance the pain relieving effects of most analgesics and is frequently combined with them in pain relief products. It may also be used to counteract the drowsiness-inducing potential of other drugs, especially antihistamines. **Pregnant women:** no evidence of risk, but crosses placenta. **Nursing mothers:** no evidence of risk to infant, but passes into breast milk. **Seniors:** no special problems. **Drug interactions:** use with care if you are also taking heart, psychological, or kidney drugs.

Stimulant/Alertness Enhancer

FIRST (ONLY) CHOICE

Generic name: Caffeine

Dose: 100 mg

Brand names: Caffedrine Capsules, Dexitac Capsules, NoDoz Tablets, Quick-Pep Tablets, Summit, Tirend Tablets, Vivarin Tablets, Wakoz

Reasons: The only choice in this category, caffeine, is an effective and useful drug for increasing alertness, reducing drowsiness, and generally improving many central nervous system functions.

Cautions: Due to excessive use of caffeine and its accessibility in coffee, soft drinks, and numerous drugs, the effects are decreased. Overdoses are also a problem because the drug is found in so many commonly used beverages and drugs.

9

Women's Special
Needs

This chapter addresses the special needs of women, for self-treatment of symptoms involving their reproductive organs and hormonal cycle. A large number of women suffer from a variety of symptoms unique to the menstrual cycle, which can be very distressing and uncomfortable. Pain associated with menstruation is reported in about half of all girls beginning menstruation, and by age 18 nearly 80% experience pain with their periods, at least occasionally, and about half of them routinely. The most common symptoms, breast pain and bloating, are usually not too severe and can be treated quite successfully. About 10% of women experience severe PMS (premenstrual syndrome), including symptoms of depression, anger, sudden bouts of tearfulness, food cravings, and headaches. The pains can be most effectively treated using the oral analgesic *ibuprofen* (see Chapter 2, page 21). Other symptoms are somewhat more difficult to deal with effectively. The symptoms of weight gain or bloating (swelling or edema) are less well treated with over-the-counter agents, but some relief can be achieved if the best agent and optimal doses of the drugs are used.

Recurrent vaginal yeast infections are common for a number of women and can be treated effectively with agents recently changed from prescription-only to over-the-counter status. For feminine hygiene, the use of douches can effectively counter complaints of odor or irritation. Simple external itching or irritation of the vaginal area can be treated using several products, which can simply relieve the symptoms, or provide anti-inflammatory effects. Products for all these indications are discussed in the following sections.

Premenstrual Syndrome, Cramps, and Pain

Crying jags, eating binges, anxiety, bloating, and some 150 other symptoms have been attributed to the week preceding a menstrual cycle. More than one-half of all women suffer routine pain at this point in their cycle, and 10% can't function normally without treatment. There is no known cause and no ready cure for this problem. Clearly, though, it's not psychological. Many theories have been proposed, but none proven, as to the source and nature of the processes causing the symptoms. Many things have been tried, but only the symptomatic treatments have been partially successful. The problems most often treated, bloating and breast pain, are usually those that are easiest to tolerate. In addition to the medications described on the next few pages, the other measures that have been found effective include eating small frequent meals, exercising, reducing salt and caffeine intake. Taking ibuprofen early, at the first onset of symptoms, seems to result in shorter and less troublesome periods.

The cause of menstrual cramps is also unknown. As with PMS, many authorities feel that exercise is beneficial for the symptoms of menstruation, and that small frequent meals reduce problems by leveling out the up and down swings in blood sugar caused by larger, spaced meals. In addition to taking specific medication for the symptoms, as described below, you will find the following helpful: avoid salty foods; reduce your sugar intake; avoid alcohol; and if you suffer from anxiety, tender breasts, or fatigue, reducing caffeine intake may help. It is also clear that get-ting an adequate amount of sleep will help to reduce menstrual symptoms.

Active Ingredients for
Menstrual Symptoms

Ibuprofen. Ibuprofen is a pain reliever and fever reducer that has been shown to be quite effective for menstrual symptoms. Many women report shorter periods, as well as less pain, when they start taking this drug at the first sign of pain. This is true of virtually all pain—the sooner the drug is taken the better it works. Waiting means the drug has to do a much more difficult task, that of countering the pain rather than preventing it. **Pregnant women:** may cause problems (slowed delivery), but no evidence of risk. **Nursing mothers:** no evidence of risk to infant. **Seniors:** reduced dose may be desirable or increased side effects may occur. **Drug interactions:** antidiabetic agents—decreased effects; antihyperten-sive and diuretic drugs—reduced effects; anticoagulants, steroids, alcohol—increased stomach irritation.

Acetaminophen. This analgesic/antipyretic is useful for mild pain and fever reduction. It does not cause stomach upset or bleeding (aspirin does). Used for over 35 years, toxic effects are unusual when label instructions are followed, but an overdose can cause serious kidney or liver damage. **Pregnant women:** safety not established, but routinely used and no evidence of risk. **Nursing mothers:** no evidence of risk to infant, but passes into breast milk. **Seniors:** no special problems. **Drug interactions:** alcohol—heavy drinking increases risk of liver damage.

Aspirin. Used for over 90 years, aspirin reduces pain and fever and has other useful effects, including reducing inflammation and preventing blood clots. It is present in many combination drugs for colds, menstrual discomfort, and other illnesses. It tends to irritate the stomach and even may cause bleeding (ulcers). **Preg-nant women:** not usually recommended, but it is frequently used (its use should be avoided if possible). **Nursing mothers:** not usu-ally recommended, frequently used, but passes into breast milk. **Seniors:** no special problems. **Drug interactions:** alcohol—in-creased risk of stomach irritation and ulcers; anti-coagulants—al-tered blood clotting time; steroids—increased stomach irritation.

Menstrual Cramps (Oral Treatment for Pain)

FIRST CHOICE

Generic name: Ibuprofen

Dose: 200–400 mg

Brand names: Addaprin, Advil, Genpril, Haltran, Medipren, Motrin IB, Nuprin, Ultraprin, Valprin

Reasons: Although ibuprofen is somewhat more expensive than aspirin or acetaminophen, it is the most effective drug in this class and is safer than aspirin. Take it with meals to reduce stomach upset (if it occurs). It has been shown to be particularly useful for cramps and pain associated with menstruation.

Cautions: Ibuprofen may cause stomach upset and ulcers (like aspirin). It is not recommended if you are pregnant or breast feeding. Patients with kidney disease should consult a physician before using these products. Ibuprofen may interact with anti-hypertensive (blood pressure) drugs, diuretics (water pills), alcohol, antacids, and anticoagulants. Consult your doctor if you take these medications.

Menstrual Cramps (Oral Treatment for Pain)

SECOND CHOICE

Generic name: Aspirin

Dose: 325–850 mg

Brand names: Anacin, Bayer Aspirin, Ecotrin, Empirin, Norwich Aspirin, St. Joseph Aspirin

Reasons: Aspirin is the standard for pain relief and fever reduction. It is also very inexpensive and is anti-inflammatory. Aspirin causes more stomach upset (nausea and vomiting) and has a higher potential for causing ulcers than ibuprofen, which makes it less desirable overall. Risks of overdose are also more significant with aspirin.

Cautions: Thousands of cases of overdose with aspirin occur each year because people do not respect this drug for what it really is—a potent, effective drug with significant toxicity. They take it in larger doses and more frequently than they should. Heavy use causes significant damage to the stomach lining (ulcers) and may also result in nutrient depletion (especially iron). It interacts with antidiabetic drugs and anticoagulants (blood thinners). **Pregnant women:** not usually recommended. **Nursing mothers:** aspirin passes into the milk. **Seniors:** no special problems.

Water Retention, Swelling, and Bloating

Although the exact cause and mechanism of water retention during the week or so before the menstrual flow begins are not known, it is a frequent problem. It may be related to hormonal changes that cause retention of sodium (salt); and with the additional salt, more water is retained as well. A reduction in the intake of salt before and during the week of menstruation may be beneficial. If these measures are not sufficient, mild diuretics (water pills) are available over the counter, which may help. The headaches, irritability, and other emotional changes may also be related to the retention of excess water (in the brain). Analgesics may also help to relieve these additional symptoms.

Active Ingredients for Water Retention

Pamabrom. This drug is a mild diuretic (a "water pill," which increases urine flow). It is related to caffeine (which also has diuretic effects and can be used for this purpose). It is used in many menstrual and PMS products. It is quite safe and does not have many undesirable side effects. In some products the dose is too low to be effective, so if the diuretic effect is needed to reduce bloating or edema (swelling), a preparation with an adequate dose of pamabrom should be selected. The biggest effect occurs during the first hour after taking the drug, but it continues for several hours more at a lower rate. **Pregnant women:** no data. **Nursing mothers:** no data. **Seniors:** no data. **Drug interactions:** none reported.

Ammonium chloride. A weak diuretic, this drug can help take off excess water that causes bloating. It is not very widely used, in part because a rather large dose is required, but mainly because of additional effects it has on the acidity of urine and blood. It is a reasonable alternative if pamabrom is not effective. **Pregnant women:** no evidence of risk. **Nursing mothers:** no data. **Seniors:** no data. **Drug interactions:** none reported.

Caffeine. Caffeine is primarily used for its stimulant effects, but it also has diuretic activity (decreases water retention). Unfortunately, the stimulant effects may be unpleasant or may even increase the severity of some menstrual symptoms, while benefiting others. A rather large dose is required to realize good diuretic activity, so it is not a preferred agent. **Pregnant women:** no evidence of risk, but crosses placenta. **Nursing mothers:** no evidence of risk to infant, but passes into breast milk. **Seniors:** no special problems. **Drug interactions:** heart and psychological drugs—use with caution.

Menstrual Cramps with Bloating

FIRST CHOICE

Take ibuprofen (above) for pain and cramps. For swelling take:

Generic name: Pamabrom *or* ammonium chloride *or* caffeine

Dose: Pamabrom, 25–50 mg; ammonium chloride, 325–650 mg; caffeine, 100–200 mg

Brand names: Aqua-Ban, Aqua-Ban Plus, Fluidex with Pamabrom, Odrinil

Reasons: One of these combinations gives you the maximum benefit from over-the-counter treatment. Ibuprofen is the best analgesic, and the diuretic agents are generally equal in their effects and safety profile. If these agents do not provide sufficient relief, dietary or other measures (described above), or a specific diagnostic workup for the problem is needed.

Cautions: Although not as powerful as prescription diuretics, these products, in conjunction with ibuprofen and the additional diet and exercise recommended, should provide the desired relief. These products have been used for many years and by large numbers of women and found to be very safe when used as directed. In the case of caffeine, since many people have a large intake in their diets (coffee, soft drinks, analgesic combinations with caffeine, and so on), an inventory of such use should be taken before caffeine is used for this purpose, or an overdose is likely.

Menstrual Cramps with Bloating

SECOND CHOICE

Combination agents with acetaminophen and a diuretic:

Generic name: Acetominophen *and* pamabrom. (Most also have an antihistamine—pyrilamine maleate—not shown to be effective or useful.)

Dose: Acetaminophen, 325–1,000 mg; pamabrom, 25–50 mg

Brand names: Bayer Select Menstrual, Midol PMS, Multi-Symptom Menstrual Discomfort Relief Formula, Pamprin, Pamprin Extra Strength, Pamprin Maximum, Premsyn PMS, Sunril

Reasons: There aren't many choices left when you get to this level, and virtually all of the available products copy each other. The acetaminophen is effective for relief of pain (but is not as good as ibuprofen), and pamabrom is as good a diuretic (water reducer) as you can get over the counter. The antihistamine may help a little by making you drowsy, but the benefit has not been shown in objective testing of these combination drugs.

Cautions: As with all combination agents, you are taking several drugs, only one of which you may need, and the others may or may not help. In this case the extra, unnecessary drug is an antihistamine, which may induce drowsiness, making it unwise to drive or do other tasks requiring alertness.

Personal Hygeine—Douche

Douching is not required to maintain good health or hygiene, but it is commonly used by some women to prevent odor. Most authorities recommend douching no more than once a week. Many prepared douches are no better than what can be simply and cheaply made at home by adding vinegar to water. Some douche preparations have special fragrances that can create problems if you should become allergic to them. Most also contain preservatives to which you may become allergic from repeated or heavy use. If vaginal discomfort (itching) or discharge is the motive for douching, it is better to determine the source of the problem so that it can be treated specifically with the appropriate antibiotic or other therapy. In the case of candida (yeast) infections, over-the-counter agents are available to effectively treat this problem. Antifungals can also be used specifically. Nonspecific antimicrobial douches (to reduce bacteria, yeast, and so on) are available and may relieve symptoms. They contain *povidone-iodine*, or other agents (not as effective), which can cure, or at least suppress, other minor infections. However, since the diagnosis is not easy to make, a physician should be consulted.

Active Ingredients in Douches

Povidone-iodine. This bactericidal agent has a broad antibiotic effect, including antiyeast and antitrichomonal activity. It is very useful as a general antibiotic for vaginal use when some minor irritation or infection is present. It has low toxicity and provides good relief in most instances. **Pregnant women:** no evidence of risk. **Nursing mothers:** no evidence of risk to infant. **Seniors:** no special problems. **Drug interactions:** due to topical use, very low risk—none reported.

For Douching (Antimicrobial)

FIRST CHOICE

Generic name: Povidone-iodine

Strength: 0.3 % conc.

Brand names: ACU-dyne Douche, Betadine Douche, Femidine Douche, Massengill Medicated Disposable Douche,

Massengill Medicated Liquid, Operand Douche, Summer's Eve Medicated Disposable Douche

Reasons: The antimicrobial activity of povidone-iodine makes these products ideal to treat minor irritation and provide the cleansing and freshening effects desired from a douche. Used as directed, these products are effective and safe. If they prove inadequate, a doctor can determine the nature of the problem and recommend appropriate therapy.

Cautions: This and all medications should not be used if you are allergic to the ingredients. If you have a reaction to the product or if the problem is not resolved within the specified time, discontinue use immediately. These products are safe when used as directed. Povidone-iodine can even be used by pregnant women when needed.

For Douching

SECOND CHOICE

Generic name: Vinegar and water

Dose: 1 tablespoon/quart

Brand names: Make your own, or Feminique Vinegar & Water Disposable, Massengill Vinegar & Water Disposable Douche (also extra mild), New Freshness Disposable Douche, Summer's Eve Vinegar & Water Disposable Douche

Reasons: These products, or making your own douche with vinegar and water provide the cleansing and freshening effect desired in most cases and are safe and easy to use. If irritation is present, or if the problem persists, a proper diagnosis should be sought. Frequent douching is not encouraged, for the reasons listed at the beginning of this section.

Cautions: As with any treatment, be sure to use the product correctly and appropriately. There are no special precautions or problems to watch for these products.

Vaginal/Labial Itching and Irritation

Inflammation of the vulva or labia of the vaginal area may result from many different causes, including trauma and mechanical or chemical irritation such as tight clothing, contamination by urine, vaginal or fecal secretions, and so on. Local allergic reactions to many agents may also cause these symptoms. For minor irritations, soreness, redness, or itching, hydrocortisone cream is one of the best treatment measures. Immediate relief may also be obtained with local anesthetics applied directly to the affected area. Cold compresses or sitz baths (sitting in warm water, often with salts added) can also provide rapid but temporary relief. The area should be cleaned thoroughly and kept dry and clean. Loose clothing should be worn to foster resolution of the inflammation and expedite healing.

Active Ingredients for Vaginal Irritation

Hydrocortisone. This drug is actually a hormone produced naturally by the body, which has potent anti-inflammatory effects. It is used topically to relieve itching and irritation, but the effects do not occur quickly. A day or so may be required to be completely effective. **Pregnant women:** no evidence of risk. **Nursing mothers:** no evidence of risk to infant. **Seniors:** reduced dose may be desirable to limit possibility of skin thinning if used for long period. **Drug interactions:** due to topical use, very low risk.

External Vaginal (Labial) Itching (From Irritation, Anti-inflammatory Therapy)

FIRST CHOICE

Generic name: Hydrocortisone

Dose: 0.5–1% conc.

Creams: Anusol HC-1, Bactine, CaldeCORT, Cortaid, Cortef Feminine Itch Cream, Cortizone-5, Dermtex HC, Dermolate,

Foille-Cort, Gynecort Creme, H2 Cort, Hydrocortisone, Hydro-Tex, Hytone, Lanacort, Pharmacort, Preparation HC, Racet SE, Rhulicort

Lotions: Cortaid, Delacort, Dermacort, Hydrocortisone, Rhulicort

Ointments: Cortaid, Cortizone-5

Sprays: Cortaid

Reasons: Hydrocortisone is truly a miracle drug, having many useful anti-inflammatory effects. It reduces itching and helps control many other symptoms. The effect is not rapid in onset, and consistent use is needed for maximum benefit. Using hydrocortisone several times a day for the first day or two will produce a more rapid effect. After that, once a day use is just as effective as multiple uses and lowers the risk of side effects.

Cautions: Excessive use of hydrocortisone preparations can lead to problems locally or, in extreme cases, even to general toxic effects, if too much is absorbed. When used topically, thinning of the skin (which can be permanent) is the most serious problem, and some increased susceptibility to infection (especially if the skin is broken) may result. When used as directed on the label, these products are some of the safest and most effective agents available for over-the-counter use.

Active Ingredient for Vaginal Itching (Symptom Relief Only)

Benzocaine. Introduced 85 years ago, benzocaine is one of the first local anesthetics. It is used in many diverse formulations for surface pain relief and also for itching. It is very poorly absorbed through the skin and mucous membranes, thereby making it quite safe for use. It has few adverse effects, though occasionally a person may become allergic to it. **Pregnant women:** no evidence of risk. **Nursing mothers:** no evidence of risk to infant. **Seniors:** no special problems. **Drug interactions:** due to topical use, very low risk—none reported.

External Vaginal (Labial) Itching (Symptom Relief Only, Topical Anesthetic)

FIRST CHOICE

Generic name: Benzocaine

Dose: 15–20% conc.

Brand names: Americaine, Benzocaine, Benzocol, Bicozene, Dermoplast, Foille, Lagol, Lanacane, Medicone Dressing, Solarcaine, Sting Kill (swabs), Sting Relief

Reasons: Benzocaine is a safe and effective local anesthetic that can deaden the symptoms of itch or pain for a short time. It has no curative effects, but merely reduces the discomfort while healing takes place. The area should be cleaned well and steps taken to reduce any irritation that may be present.

Cautions: Since these products have no curative effects, the source of the problem is not corrected. They are for temporary use only. If an infection or other cause is identified, it must be treated and/or corrective action taken to prevent reoccurrences or worsening of the problem, which may occur if the symptoms are suppressed.

Vaginal Candidiasis

Candida is a yeast (a small plant-like organism that grows in warm, moist environments), which is a normal inhabitant of our bodies and only becomes a problem when it gets out of control. The checks and balances of our bodies usually keep it at a low level, but sometimes it proliferates and causes symptoms of candidiasis. This occurs especially when antibacterial therapy (antibiotics) is given, since normal bacteria serve to keep the yeast population under control.

   Until recently, the only effective treatment was available exclusively by prescription. However, because some women have recurrent problems with candida, and two of the antibiotics used to treat this problem are deemed safe and effective in curing this infection, the drugs are now available over the counter. In order to be sure the infection is candida (there are 150 candida strains, but only 10 are thought to induce the infection), it is best to have it diagnosed by a physician. If the same symptoms reoccur, they can then be self-treated. In addition to using the medications as described, loose cotton garments should be worn and occlusive underwear or pantihose abandoned. Eating yogurt (natural, nonpasteurized) has also been helpful in controlling the infection by reestablishing normal flora.

Active Ingredients for Candidiasis

Clotrimazole. An antibiotic used for yeast and fungal infections, clotrimazole is effective for athlete's foot, jock itch, ringworm, diaper rash, oral candida (or thrush), and vaginal candida infections. Used since 1976, it is applied topically to the site. Adverse effects are quite rare, but some people may have burning or irritation at the site of application. **Pregnant women:** no evidence of risk. **Nursing mothers:** no evidence of risk. **Seniors:** no special needs or cautions. **Drug interactions:** none reported.

Miconazole. Miconazole is the other widely used, effective antifungal/antiyeast agent, which has been in use since the 1970s. It is also useful for all of the indications noted above for clotrimazole. The two drugs really cannot be distinguished from one another in the therapy of these indications. Side effects are quite rare. **Pregnant women:** no evidence of risk. **Nursing mothers:** no evidence of risk. **Seniors:** no special needs or cautions. **Drug interactions:** none reported.

Vaginal Itching/Candidiasis (Antiyeast/Antifungal, Topical Treatment)

FIRST CHOICE

Generic names: Clotrimazole *or* miconazole

Dose: Clotrimazole, 1% cream or 100 mg tablets; miconazole, 2% cream or 100 or 200 mg tablets

Brand names: Femcare (cream and tablets), Gyne-Lotrimin (cream and tablets), Mycelex-7 (cream and tablets), Monistat 7

Reasons: Both clotrimazole and miconazole are very effective and safe for topical use. They are really equal in most respects. There is some price competition now, so look for the best deal.

Cautions: Side effects are very rare with these drugs and when used as directed should not cause any problems. They are nearly always effective in curing the infection.

10

Nutrition and Weight Control

Between one-third and one-half of the U.S. population take vitamin and mineral supplements; yet little is known about their long-term health benefits or the possible consequences of using the frequently very high doses that many people take. The human body's need for vitamins and minerals was discovered about 1500 B.C., when it was noted that certain diseases could be cured by eating a particular food. Scientific experimentation then showed that dietary deficiencies in animals could produce diseases, and the vitamin and mineral deficiencies responsible for particular diseases were identified and characterized. Biochemical functions were later established for many vitamins and minerals, and the dose requirements to prevent disease were determined. Today we are in the process of discovering new, additional biochemical functions for vitamins and minerals, with the suspected potential for going beyond just health main- tenance to disease prevention. The traditional view of vitamins as being essential for preventing deficiency diseases and serving as enzymes or catalysts has held up well for decades, but additional roles as protective agents for a wide range of illnesses have been proposed. While it is well beyond the scope of this book to discuss each of the individual vitamins and minerals and the state of scientific evidence concerning their effects and potential benefits, this chapter provides a brief recounting of the current understanding and some recommendations for their use.

The other topic of this chapter concerns weight control. Individuals weighing significantly more than their ideal weight (based on age, sex, height, and frame size) are at risk of major health problems. The most significant problems relate to the heart (it works too hard), sleep apnea (breathing stops at night), other gland dysfunctions (such as diabetes), and osteoarthritis (joint problems). Other problems, including hypertension (high blood pressure), increased risk of sudden death from heart attacks, strokes, and atherosclerosis, are also more common in obese people. These are the health reasons for losing excess pounds. In addition, our society places great emphasis on how people look, which makes it difficult for overweight people. Weight loss is achieved either by reducing food intake or increasing physical activity or, preferably, both. There are no magic formulas or potions. Many "fad" diets have been developed and tried by millions, but they only work for a few—nearly always as a direct result of reducing the overall calorie intake of the individual. As it happens, a particular food type or regimen—or the "hype"—gets certain people motivated to make it happen, when they may have tried many others previously without success. When dieting, a healthy state must be maintained by providing the necessary building blocks (vitamins and minerals), while reducing the total caloric intake. This can be accomplished many ways, including some help from drugs or fillers or low and noncalorie-containing sugar and fat substitutes. Recommendations for the most effective over-the-counter agents in this class are described next.

Diet Aids

Both artificial sweeteners and appetite suppressants are popular agents in the battle to lose and control weight. There is only one over-the-counter drug recognized as safe and effective for suppressing the appetite, and it is not terribly effective (but can help some). The drug, phenylpropanolamine, is frequently used as a nasal decongestant and even has some stimulant effects (similar to caffeine). As a side effect, it reduces appetite in some people. It is effective for several hours, and is commonly used in conjunction with another drug that adds bulk to the stomach by swelling when combined with water (or other liquids) or with caffeine to help stimulate mood and energy level.

Active Ingredients in Appetite Suppressants

Phenylpropanolamine. Phenylpropanolamine is a widely used decongestant that shrinks blood vessels. A side effect, appetite suppression, makes this drug the only over-the-counter diet aid available. It is likely to produce undesirable effects, including increased heart rate, raised blood pressure, palpitations, and sleep disruption, when used in optimal doses. **Pregnant women:** safety not established, possible problems but no evidence of risk. **Nursing mothers:** passes into milk. **Seniors:** decrease dose or increased side effects likely. **Drug interactions:** antihypertensives—decreased effects; MAOI (monoamine oxidase inhibitor) drugs (certain antidepressants)—risk of acute hypertension (high blood pressure).

Methylcellulose. This commonly used agent has been widely used as a laxative (bulk producing, softening agent) for over 40 years. It is not absorbed, but acts in the stomach to absorb water and provide bulk and volume to give the sensation of "fullness." It needs to be taken with adequate amounts of water to be most effective. **Pregnant women:** no evidence of risk. **Nursing mothers:** no evidence of risk. **Seniors:** no special needs or cautions. **Drug interactions:** may interfere with absorption of other drugs.

Caffeine. This naturally occurring drug is found in several plants and is used very widely for its stimulatory effects. Additional effects of this drug include stimulation of water loss by effects on the kidney, stimulation of the heart muscle, and relaxation of smooth muscle. It has also been shown to enhance the pain relieving effects of most analgesics and is frequently combined with them in pain relief products. In the case of diet aids, it is used for its mood elevating and fatigue relieving effects to help deter the hungry, depressed dieter from eating to relieve these symptoms. **Pregnant women:** no evidence of risk. **Nursing mothers:** no evidence of risk. **Seniors:** no special needs or cautions. **Drug interactions:** heart drugs, psychological drugs—use with caution.

Appetite Suppressants with Bulk Producer (Oral Use)

FIRST CHOICE

Generic name: Phenylpropanolamine (appetite suppressant) *and* methylcellulose (bulk producer)

Dose: 75 mg

Brand names: Acutrim 16 Hour Steady Control Tablets, Acutrim Late Day Tablets, Acutrim II Maximum Strength Tablets, Dieutrim T.D. (Some have local anesthetics added, however they have not been shown to be effective.)

Reasons: Hunger is registered and monitored in several ways, including determining whether the stomach is empty and whether the appropriate amounts of energy-producing materials are in the blood. For better results, the appetite suppressing drug can be combined with a bulk producer with no calories that can help make the stomach "feel" as though it has food in it. The ingredients used in these products are fiber-type materials which, when taken with sufficient water, expand in the stomach to produce bulk and help alleviate the empty feeling. Phenylpro- panolamine is a mild appetite suppressant that helps reduce food intake by curbing the appetite.

Cautions: These products can cause several different problems, including those resulting from the direct side effects of the appetite suppressant: excitement, nervousness, and increased blood pressure, for example. The bulk producing agent can also cause problems if the material is taken as a pill and is not swallowed completely before water begins to swell it into the bulky material.

Many of these products are consumed as liquids or "shakes," thus avoiding this problem. If the swelling takes place while the pill is in the throat, the result is a very unpleasant or painful effect. For these reasons, take care using these agents and follow directions carefully.

Appetite Suppressants with Caffeine (Oral Use)

SECOND CHOICE

Generic name: Phenylpropanolamine (appetite suppressant) *and* caffeine (stimulant)

Dose: Phenylpropanolamine, 37.5–75 mg; caffeine, 100–140 mg

Brand names: Prolamine Capsules, Thinz-Back-To-Nature, Thinz-Span

Reasons: Two of the natural consequences of dieting (eating less, even when accompanied by an increase in exercise) are to have less energy and to have mood swings (mild depression). Both of these effects can be at least partially countered by taking advantage of the stimulant effects of caffeine, thereby helping you stay on the diet, eat less, and be more active.

Cautions: Since both of these drugs can have stimulatory effects on the nervous system, increased blood pressure, nervousness, and excitement may occur. Persons having medical conditions that might be made worse by such effects (high blood pressure and nervous conditions, for example) should avoid these combination products. If you drink a lot of coffee or cola drinks, your caffeine intake may already be so high that no further effects, except toxicity, will result if you use these products. They are most effective in persons not routinely using, or currently restricting, caffeine.

Appetite Suppressants Alone (Oral Use)

THIRD CHOICE

Generic name: Phenylpropanolamine

Dose: 5–75 mg

Brand names: Appedrine Tablets, Control, Dex-A-Diet Extended Release/Maximum Strength, Dexatrim Capsules/Maximum Strength, Dexatrim Pre-Meal, Phenoxine, Super Odrinex, Thinz Before Meals, Unitrol

Reasons: There is only one over-the-counter drug that has been shown effective and safe for appetite suppression. This effect is not very strong and is less effective alone than with a combination adding a bulk producer (to help fill an empty stomach) or a stimulant (caffeine), to increase the depressed energy level and mood. In addition, many of these drugs contain such a low level of the appetite suppressant that little or no benefit is obtained.

Cautions: This drug is a decongestant with one of its side effects being appetite suppression. For this reason, doses must be followed as directed on the label, and people with high blood pressure should not take this drug. Excitement, nervousness, agitation, and sleeplessness may result from taking this drug.

Ingredients in Artificial Sweeteners

Aspartame (Equal). Aspartame is an artificial sweetener, which has very few calories, and yet is so sweet that virtually no calories are ingested in a normal serving. It is used in soft drinks and many other foods as a diet aid to reduce the number of calories. Due to loss of sweetness at high temperatures, it cannot be used in many foods. It has been voluntarily consumed by more people than any other synthetic chemical in history. It does help to reduce the total calorie intake if users do not eat more, substituting products with aspartame for things they would not have eaten anyway. It has a very sweet taste (200 times that of sugar for the same amount) and lacks the unpleasant aftertaste frequently associated with saccharin. Some have claimed that hunger is actually increased by the intake of aspartame, but objective, scientific investigations have failed to support this claim. Most tests have shown either a decrease in hunger or no change. Even with high doses, no accumulation of this sweetener is seen in the body and, despite claims to the contrary by some, no definite symptom complex has been connected with aspartame use. It is considered safe for use by all segments of the population (young and old). As with all such aids, aspartame can be most useful if used as part of a program to reduce caloric intake in a complete diet and exercise program to reduce weight or maintain a desired weight. If the consumption of low-calorie foods is used as an excuse to eat a high-calorie food, or if the intake of food is not restricted, daily total calorie intake may remain unchanged and no weight loss will occur.

Saccharin (Necta Sweet, Sweeta). This artificial, nonnutritive (no calories) sweetener has been the center of controversy for many years. It was discovered in 1879 and has been used for many years by those desiring to reduce caloric intake. Several different toxic effects have been attributed to saccharin, most recently the scare concerning the potential cancer-causing effects. In rats given high doses of saccharin for long periods of time, increased urinary bladder cancer was noted. However, no such effects were seen in other animals, including mice, hamsters, or monkeys, and no connection to human bladder cancer has been found. Recent studies suggest that a unique feature in rats makes them susceptible, while no other species are at risk. As with all health considerations, the possible risks must be weighed against the benefits. If the use of this artificial, nonnutritive sweetener benefits the person (such as in diabetes or in weight reduction) more than the risk (in this case infinitesimally small), then the product should be available and be used properly for its intended and proven effects.

Vitamin and Mineral Supplements

Unfortunately, data collected to date have not shown any dramatic effects for the millions of people taking vitamin and mineral supplements. The risk of mortality for regular users of supplements is, so far, similar to that for nonusers, suggesting no pronounced ill effects or dramatic positive benefits either. There is also no evidence of increased longevity among vitamin and mineral supplement users. However, many people, including some famous and well-known scientists, have claimed significant benefits and encouraged the use of mega doses of certain vitamins and minerals. On the other hand, many people are also concerned about the risks of toxicity associated with the "overuse" of these agents by those who ingest certain nutrients in doses much larger than what has been determined to be the official "recommended daily allowance" (RDA).

Entire books have been written on the potential benefits and curative effects of vitamins, minerals, and other supplements. But those that are scientifically sound and valid clearly indicate that we don't know the answers. Many suggested and possible benefits have been pointed out or postulated, but the data just are not there to document these effects. While it is true that when we are ill or under stress, we clearly need more than the usual amounts, how much and what kind is not evident. The B complex of vitamins is generally recognized as being useful and needed in extra quantities at such times, but how much is not as widely accepted.

Vitamin D is clearly important for increasing calcium absorption and metabolism and may have other beneficial effects for reproductive and skin health and to prevent some cancers. Vitamin K is important also in calcium metabolism and may help prevent osteoporosis. Vitamin B6 may play a role in premenstrual syndrome, steroid actions, and immune function. The antioxidant group, including vitamins C and E and beta-carotene, may have protective effects for age-related changes, cardiovascular disease, and certain cancers. The intake and level of antioxidants in the body have been repeatedly shown to correlate with decreased heart disease; and they may have a possible protective role in certain cancers (rectal, lung, cervical, and breast primarily), but more work is needed to prove cause and effect. Many trace minerals have been suggested to have important roles in preventing various illnesses and curing some diseases, but the data necessary to draw good solid conclusions are lacking. Overall, there is data suggesting that doses of vitamins and minerals may need to be refined to include higher doses than have previously been identified as optimal for good health (the RDAs). These could reduce the risk of certain diseases that afflict our population, given our lifestyles and environmental exposures. The results of ongoing studies will be critical in determining such effects and the effective doses.

On the downside, we must keep in mind that vitamins and minerals do indeed interact with each other and with both prescription and nonprescription drugs. They may alter both the potency and the duration of effect of drugs. Particularly vitamins, but some minerals as well, can affect (most commonly) anticoagulants, anticonvulsants, antipsychotics, antibiotics, and diuretics. Too much zinc can also induce copper deficiency and anemia. Finally, it should be realized that vitamins and minerals and even food supplements and amino acids, also act like drugs, since they supply essential building blocks for the body and alter the balance of these in the system. Many such products are available, and they contain numerous ingredients and in concentrations many times higher than what we could get in our diets (even if healthy and well balanced). The real effects of such treatments, especially in high doses, are unknown. The rule of thumb should be "moderation in all things" to avoid potential consequences which too much of anything is bound to cause.

Many vitamins are dosed using the "International Units" (IU) nomenclature which is based upon the early quantitation of vitamin amounts using biological (living animal) test systems to measure activity. We now know the exact chemical structure, purity, and activity of these vitamins and could use the absolute amounts (weights), but the traditional IU designation continues to be used for both traditional and international standardization reasons.

Calcium Supplements

Calcium is the most abundant mineral in the body and makes up more than 90% of our bones and teeth. It is essential in the formation and maintenance of strong bones and teeth, for blood clotting, transmission of nerve signals, and the normal contraction of muscle. It is found in the diet primarily in milk and dairy foods, dark leafy green vegetables, dried beans, and nuts. The diet may not contain enough calcium for everyone, particularly for women during pregnancy and breast feeding. Supplements are widely available to make up for any dietary deficiency. Symptoms of deficiency do not develop until the situation is serious, because the body takes the calcium needed for other purposes from the bones, and softening of the bones may not be noticed for many years. Severe deficiency may also cause abnormal nervous system stimulation and muscle problems. Vitamin D is given along with calcium to increase the absorption and use of this mineral. Excessive calcium intake may reduce the amount of iron and zinc absorbed and cause constipation and nausea. Effects on the heart and kidneys are also seen, especially when high doses of calcium and vitamin D are ingested. To maintain optimal calcium levels, a supplemental intake of 50–100% of the RDA is a very reasonable measure. See the products listed below for the best sources of calcium to supplement your dietary intake.

Calcium Supplements (Calcium plus Vitamin D)

FIRST CHOICE

Generic name: Calcium carbonate *with* vitamin D

Dose: Calcium carbonate, 150–300 mg; vitamin D, 60–133 IU

Brand names: Calcet, Caltrate Jr., Caltro, De-Cal, Os-Cal 250+D, Oysco 'D', Oyst-Cal-D, Oystercal-D 250, Scooby-Doo Calcium Chewable

Reasons: These products contain the required calcium and the vitamin D that is necessary for complete utilization of the calcium. Other products either lack the vitamin D, or have other vitamins or minerals added. As discussed later (page 209), if additional vitamins and minerals are desired, the complete supplements are suggested, rather than the hit-or-miss approach of getting some here and there, which may lead to excess doses of some and none of others. Calcium also is available in other salt forms (like gluconate, lactate, and phosphate), but the carbonate salt is recommended as the first choice.

In a few rare instances individuals do not produce normal amounts of stomach acid (hypochlorohydria). In such cases the carbonate form of calcium does not dissolve well and cannot be absorbed. This is not a problem with the other salts (gluconate, lactate, and phosphate) which are then the best choice, although separate supplementation with vitamin D will be necessary to realize the full benefits because these forms are not manufactured with vitamin D included.

Cautions: As with all other drugs, mineral supplements must be treated sensibly. Many of them contain additional vitamins or minerals, and when taken in conjunction with others, may result in overdoses or a complete lack of essential nutrients. Therefore, if only calcium is needed, the calcium plus vitamin D preparations are recommended, but for a broader supplementation, the complete multiple vitamin or vitamin-mineral supplements are the best choice (see page 205).

Iron Supplements

Iron has a very important role in the formation of red blood cells and in the transport of oxygen throughout the body by the blood. It is also very important for a number of enzymes (the little machines that do much of the work to build, repair, and maintain the body). Dietary iron comes from meat, eggs, chicken, fish, green leafy vegetables, fruit, grain cereals, breads, nuts, and dried beans. Increased iron is required during pregnancy and for several months after childbirth. Most diets supply enough iron, but vegetarians, women with heavy menstrual periods, or people with chronic blood loss diseases (such as ulcers) may require supplementation. Iron deficiency causes anemia, the symptoms of which are pallor, fatigue, shortness of breath, and palpitations. Iron poisoning (overdose) is very dangerous, manifested by symptoms of abdominal pain, nausea, vomiting, fever, abdominal bloating, dehydration, and low blood pressure. Excessive intake of iron, especially combined with vitamin C, may cause toxic levels of iron accumulation in various organs, resulting in congestive heart failure, cirrhosis of the liver, and diabetes.

Iron Supplements

FIRST CHOICE

Generic name: Ferrous gluconate

Dose: 35–40 mg

Brand names: Fergon Elixir, Fergon Tablets, (plus several generic "ferrous gluconate" products in tablets or capsules)

Reasons: Ferrous gluconate is the easiest to absorb of the various salts of iron commercially available for the body, and has the lowest incidence of side effects (adverse taste or smell). Many of the preparations contain ferrous fumarate or ferrous sulfate, and a number also contain from two to eight additional vitamins. As discussed later in this section, more complete supplements are recommended when vitamins and or minerals are desired. The products recommended here are for use only when iron supplements alone are needed or desired.

Cautions: Many of the available iron supplements contain other vitamins or minerals and do not supply only the needed iron. Most people's diets contain sufficient amounts of these other vitamins and minerals. If a multivitamin/mineral supplement is desired to supplement an inadequate diet or as insurance for the intake of adequate amounts for good health, a complete supplement with all of the required vitamins and minerals is recommended (see below), rather than the hit-or-miss method of getting selected vitamins or minerals in varying doses. Ferrous sulfate is more commonly available than ferrous gluconate (especially in combination agents) because it is less expensive, but the gluconate form (salt) is tolerated better by most people, so is recommended as the first choice.

Multivitamin Supplements

Many people see vitamins and minerals as health insurance that is worth the cost and effort to be sure they are doing all they can to maintain optimal health. Medical scientists generally agree that taking extra vitamins does not significantly combat colds, relieve stress, boost energy, or prevent illnesses (except in cases of vitamin deficiencies—which are very rare in the United States). Most health experts agree that the recommended daily allowances for vitamins and minerals are more than sufficient for the needs of most people. However, many of the supplements are confusing, and many people think they feel better in spite of what science says about needed vitamin and mineral intake. To be sure that you are getting optimal vitamin and mineral levels, it is reasonable to take 50–100 percent of the RDA as a supplement. However, more than two out of every three supplements available have either an excess or a deficiency in their content of one or more of the required vitamins and minerals. Most have an excess, and the wasted money is the biggest concern. But since many people feel that more is better, they take these supplements even though their diet provides the recommended daily allowances. This is not a problem for most people, but it could be

New Recommended Daily Allowances (RDAs) for Vitamins and Minerals

Vitamin/Mineral	Males	Females
Vitamin A	5,000 IU	5,000 IU
Vitamin B1 (thiamine)	1.5 mg	1.5 mg
Vitamin B2 (riboflavin)	1.7 mg	1.7 mg
Vitamin B3 (niacin)	20 mg	20 mg
Vitamin B6	2.0 mg	1.6 mg
Vitamin B12	3.0 mcg	2.0 mcg
Vitamin D	400 IU	400 IU
Vitamin C	60 mg	60 mg
Vitamin E	30 IU	40 IU
Vitamin K	80 mcg	65 mcg
Folic acid	0.4 mg	0.4 mg
Biotin	0.3 mg	0.3 mg
Calcium, under 25 years	800 mg	800 mg
over 25 years	1,200 mg	1,200 mg
Iron	10 mg	15 mg
Magnesium	350 mg	280 mg
Selenium	70 mcg	55 mcg
Zinc	15 mg	12 mg

for some who take therapeutic (very high) doses (3–8 times the RDA) of one or more vitamins or minerals. Even the water soluble vitamins can cause significant problems when taken in excess. Kidney stones are a major harmful effect of mega doses of vitamin C. Overdoses of the fat-soluble vitamins can be even more dangerous, since excessive levels may build up and cause overt toxicity as well as interfere with the normal use of other essential vitamins, minerals, or other nutrients.

Multivitamin Supplements (Half the RDA)

FIRST CHOICE

Generic name: See the table on page 205 for a list of recommended daily allowances of vitamins and minerals.

Brand names: Bugs Bunny Children's Chewable Tablets, Bugs Bunny with Extra C Children's Chewable Tablets, Chew-Vites Chewable Tablets, Flintstones Children's Chewable Tablets, Flintstones with Extra C Children's Chewable Tablets, Fruity Chews Chewable Tablets, Poly-Vi-Sol Chewable Tablets, Sunkist Multis Regular, Sunkist Multis Plus C, Syrvite Liquid, Vi-Daylin Chewable Tablets, Vi-Daylin Multi-vitamin Liquid

Reasons: These products contain half of the recommended daily allowance of vitamins. This is a very reasonable dose to supplement a diet that could be inadequate in one or more of these nutrients and not cause any concern about overdosage.

Multivitamin Supplements (Full RDA)

SECOND CHOICE

Generic name: See the table on page 205 for a list of vitamins and minerals.

Brand names: Dayalets Filmtabs, One-A-Day Essential Tablets, One-A-Day Plus Extra C Tablets, One-Tablet-Daily Tablets,

Theragran Jr. Children's Chewable Tablets, Theragran Jr. Children's Chewable Tablets with Extra Vitamin C, Theragran Tablets, Unicap (capsules and tablets), Unicap Jr. Chewable Tablets, Vigran Tablets, Zymacap Capsules

Reasons: These products contain the full recommended daily allowance of vitamins for a normal healthy individual. They provide all of the normal needs and, when diet intake of vitamins is added, are more than adequate to maintain appropriate levels of all vitamins in the body. Only in special circumstances, such as illness or specific diseases of deficiency, would there be any rationale to take more. Taking more risks possible overdose, especially of those vitamins that are not water soluble and therefore not easily eliminated.

Multivitamin Supplements with Iron (Half the RDA)

FIRST CHOICE

Generic name: See the table on page 205 for a list of vitamins and minerals.

Brand names: Bugs Bunny Plus Iron Chewable Tablets, Flintstones Plus Iron Chewable Tablets, Fruity Chews with Iron Chewable Tablets, NeoVadrin Children's Chewable Tablets with Iron, Poly-Vi-Sol with Iron Chewable Tablets, Sunkist Multis Plus Iron, Vi-Daylin Plus Iron Chewable Tablets, Vi-Daylin Plus Iron Liquid

Reasons: In addition to one-half of the RDA of vitamins, these products contain iron in amounts sufficient to supplement a diet that provides inadequate amounts of iron, or for those requiring a little extra iron. Only in special cases of disease (for example, anemia or bleeding ulcers), or perhaps for some women with heavy menstrual flow or during pregnancy, is there any need for iron in amounts greater than what is supplied in these products.

Multivitamin Supplements with Iron (Full RDA)

SECOND CHOICE

Generic names: See the table on page 205 for a list of vitamins and minerals.

Brand names: Avail Tablets, Centrovite Jr. Tablets, Centrum Jr. Plus Iron Tablets, Dayalets Plus Iron Filmtabs, Femiron Tablets, Flintstones Complete Chewable Tablets, One-Tablet-Daily with Iron Tablets, Stuart Formula Tablets, Theragran Jr. with Iron Chewable Tablets, Unicap Plus Iron Tablets

Reasons: In addition to the full daily allowance of vitamins, these products contain iron in amounts sufficient to supplement a diet that provides inadequate amounts of iron, or for the needs of those requiring a little extra iron. Only in special cases of disease (for example, anemia or bleeding ulcers), or perhaps for some women with heavy menstrual flow and during pregnancy, is there any need for iron in amounts greater than are supplied in these products.

Multivitamins with Minerals (Full RDA Plus Minerals)

FIRST CHOICE

Generic name: See the table on page 205 for a list of vitamins and minerals.

Brand names: Arbon, Bugs Bunny Vitamins and Minerals Chewable Tablets, Centrum, Geritol Complete Tablets, Gevral T Tablets, Sunkist Multis Complete

Reasons: These products are very complete, containing the full daily vitamin needs and multiple minerals in adequate supplemental doses. They supply all that should normally be needed, even when the dietary intake is very low in one or more of these necessary nutrients. Only in cases of specific disease, where there could be special needs for one or another of these nutrients to correct a deficiency or treat a special problem, would there be justification for taking more than is provided in these products. In such a case, a practitioner skilled in diagnosing and treating such problems should be consulted, and the problem should be treated with specific high-potency preparations of the nutrient(s) needed.

Vitamin C

Vitamin C is essential for a variety of body activities, especially for the proper function of many enzymes. It is important for maintenance of healthy bones, teeth, gums, ligaments, blood vessels, and many body organs. Vitamin C is found in most fresh fruits and vegetables. A normal, healthy diet contains sufficient vitamin C, but it is used more rapidly after serious injury, burns, or during extremes in temperature. Supplements are often needed in smokers, the elderly, the chronically ill, and for women taking birth control pills. There is no convincing evidence that large doses prevent colds or other illnesses, but some reduction in severity of symptoms may occur. Mild deficiencies of vitamin C may cause weakness, aches and pains, swollen gums, and nose bleeds. The risk of harmful effects from taking too much are relatively low, but mega doses (more than 1 gram a day) may cause diarrhea, nausea, and stomach cramps. Kidney stones may also develop from excessive use of large doses.

Vitamin E

Vitamin E rivals vitamin C for the incidence of unfounded rumors and folklore purporting its amazing virtues to prevent or cure a variety of ills. Vitamin E is vital for healthy cell structure and for slowing the aging process and maintaining enzyme activity. It helps protect the lungs and other tissues from damage by pollutants. It helps form red blood cells and is important in the production of energy in the heart and muscles. Vegetable oils are a good source for this vitamin, as are green leafy vegetables and whole grain cereals and bread. Normal diets supply enough vitamin E. Supplements may be warranted for those consuming large amounts of polyunsaturated fats or with impaired intestinal absorption, liver disease, cystic fibrosis, and in premature infants. Harmful effects of overuse are rare, but nausea, abdominal pain, vomiting, and diarrhea may occur. Large doses may also reduce the efficient use of other important and essential vitamins (including vitamins A, D, and K).

11

Miscellaneous Disorders

This final chapter contains a discussion of several miscellaneous disorders for which over-the-counter remedies are commonly sought. Effective, accessible treatments exist for most; for some, methods of self-care remain elusive.

Aphrodisiacs

The search for agents that will improve sexual performance, or enhance the pleasure of sex, has been a never ending quest of man. Unfortunately, none of the many drugs or measures advocated has been shown to be safe and effective. Some drugs widely used for this purpose have severe toxic effects and are not recommended. Most of them have mutagenic effects (causing mutations in the offspring), as well as direct toxic effects. Many exotic agents have been claimed to possess aphrodisiacal powers, but in fact, the only real effect seems to be the enrichment of those preying on the public with these tonics, potions, and elixirs. In the best of cases, they are harmless, but in many cases there is a considerable risk associated with their use. Many millions of dollars have been spent on preparations made from animal organs or plants, which carry not only a direct toxic potential, but also may transmit viral or other microbial (bacteria, fungi, rickettsia, and so on) infections from the animal tissue source to man. Other preparations have been shown to contain anabolic steroids—the drugs (hormones) that are being used by some athletes to improve their physical performance or appearance, at considerable risk to their health.

Earwax

Normally, earwax is not a problem. However, some people produce unusually large amounts of earwax, and when it accumulates it may become dry or hard and induce some loss of hearing. Alternatively, when exposed to water (such as when swimming), it may soften and become an ideal place for bacteria to grow, resulting in swimmer's ear (an infection of the outer ear discussed later in this chapter). To remove earwax, soften it using light mineral oil or one of the products containing carbamide peroxide (listed below). Then remove it by gently washing it from the ear with water expelled from a syringe or bulb-type instrument. Never use force and never insert an instrument into the ear to remove wax. After removal, apply 70% alcohol and dry the ear thoroughly. If there has been any discharge from the ear, or if the eardrum has been perforated in the past, a physician should be consulted before attempting to remove earwax.

Active Ingredients for Earwax Removal

Carbamide peroxide. Carbamide peroxide is a topical agent used to soften earwax. It also has anti-infective properties, acting as an antiseptic to help reduce the possibility of infection in the outer ear. **Pregnant women:** no evidence of risk. **Nursing mothers:** no evidence of risk. **Seniors:** no special needs or cautions. **Drug interactions:** due to topical use, very low risk—none reported.

Earwax Removal (Topical Use)

FIRST (ONLY) CHOICE *adults, seniors, children, infants*

Generic name: Carbamide peroxide

Dose: See label

Brand names: Aurocaine Ear Drops, Auro Ear Drops, Debrox Drops, E.R.O., Murine Ear Wax Removal System and Ear Drops, Otix Ear Drops

Reasons: There is only one ear ingredient recognized as both safe and effective for the removal of earwax, and it is the active ingredient in the products listed. The other products in this category contain ingredients that will be withdrawn from the market in the near future. They will switch to this ingredient or not be available any longer.

Cautions: Do not be overly vigorous in the physical manipulations used to remove the softened wax. Rough procedures can damage or break the eardrum. The wax should be removed only by rinsing with water under gentle pressure.

Hiccups

Most of us have experienced the transient, benign annoyance of hiccups. The cause of hiccups has not been determined, and no useful function has been attributed to this phenomenon. Not only people, but various other animals are known to experience hiccups; even babies in the womb may have bouts of hiccups. There is no clear male or female preponderance, nor any social, racial, geographic, or other stratification in their occurrence. Various causes have been associated with hiccups, including excessive food or alcohol intake and sudden changes in temperature. Treatment of hiccups is more art than science. No drug is universally effective, nor are the myriad home remedies always effective. Among the more successful measures are gargling with water, sipping ice water, swallowing granulated sugar, and biting on a lemon. Perhaps the best known is breathing into a paper bag. No firm advice can be given for this affliction. Just try one or two remedies, and chances are they will go away.

Poisoning

Poisoning is a frequent and widespread problem, for which the best measures are prevention, prevention, and more prevention. However, when poisoning occurs, treatment must be prompt for maximum effectiveness. For the vast majority of drugs and other chemicals involved in poisonings, there is no specific treatment or antidote. Minimizing the length of exposure and promptly treating the symptoms are the highest priorities. Because not all poisonings should be dealt with in the same manner, it is best to have the phone number of a poison control center handy, or get it and call them immediately for instructions in an emergency. You will need to identify the agent and the amount ingested if at all possible. The center will then advise you on what to administer, if anything, and whether to induce vomiting. Having ipecac syrup on hand if vomiting is advised saves valuable time (from 30 minutes to 2 hours usually) and may even prevent the need for emergency medical treatment.

Active Ingredient for Poisoning

Ipecac syrup. Ipecac has been used for many years as the emetic of choice to induce vomiting in both adult and pediatric patients. For drug overdose, and for many other types of poison ingestion, ipecac is very effective in emptying the stomach contents, thereby stopping the further exposure and increased absorption of the poison into the body. Ipecac induces vomiting in more than 90% of patients, and the frequency of adverse side effects is very low. Only very rarely are serious complications seen. It is safe for home administration, and having it at home saves valuable time in treating poisoning cases. To obtain the best advice on what to do in case of poisoning, consult a poison control center by telephone for instructions specific to the ingested agent. If instructed to induce vomiting, give ipecac syrup. It usually acts within 15–30 minutes, and can be readministered if it doesn't work the first time. It is a local irritant to the stomach, and also triggers a central vomiting reflex to hasten emptying of the stomach.

Poisoning (To Induce Vomiting)

FIRST (ONLY) CHOICE

Generic name: Ipecac syrup

Dose: See label

Brand names: Ipecac syrup

Reasons: This is the most useful and reliable method to induce vomiting. It acts quite rapidly (15–30 minutes), and effectively empties the stomach to remove the poison and prevent further entrance of the poison into the blood. A glass of water should be given after administration of ipecac to obtain best results.

Cautions: Ipecac is generally very safe and effective, without complications. If vomiting does not occur, and especially if repeated doses are administered, toxic effects on the heart are possible, so consideration should be given to removing it from the stomach (consult a doctor or poison control center).

Swimmer's Ear

This infection of the external ear canal may occur when water washes away the protective earwax and allows an infection to develop, or when excess earwax becomes a breeding ground for germs. Unfortunately, there are no products available over the counter for treating this infection, and you must see a doctor to get an antibiotic. It can be prevented by using earplugs if you are prone to this problem, and also by being careful to dry the ear after swimming or engaging in other activities where water gets in the ears.

Teeth Desensitizers

These products consist of a group of toothpastes that can be used to help reduce sensitivity of teeth to heat and cold. Review of these products has shown that they are effective and safe. There are two ingredients (*potassium nitrate* and *strontium chloride*) that in clinical testing have been shown to be effective tooth desensitizers. Only one has been formally approved as effective by the USFDA (potassium nitrate) and the other is still pending approval, but both are recognized as safe by the USFDA. The mechanism(s) of how they work is not known, but the best theories include a direct effect on plugging small tubules in the tooth dentin to reduce access to the tooth nerve, and a direct effect on the nerves themselves to reduce sensitivity.

Teeth Desensitizers

FIRST (ONLY) CHOICE

Generic name: Potassium nitrate

Dose: 5%

Brand names: Aquafresh Sensitive, Crest Sensitivity Protection, Denquel, Mint Sensodyne, Promise

Reasons: These products contain the only ingredient recognized safe and effective to reduce the sensitivity of teeth to heat and cold.

Cautions: None of any concern.

Teeth Whiteners

The quest for a brighter, more attractive smile has fueled rapid growth for teeth whiteners. These products attract the attention of appearance-conscious consumers. There's no doubt that they do work, especially on mild or moderate stains. The question is whether they are safe. The answer isn't totally clear yet, but when properly used, any risk would appear to be quite low. The USFDA has recently ruled that these products are drugs rather than cosmetic products and therefore must be approved for use. They have been ordered removed from the market until such approval is granted or unless a court appeal changes the ruling. They may or may not be available depending on the progress of these proceedings. (Brands remain available without the active ingredients.)

Teeth Whiteners

FIRST (ONLY) CHOICE

Generic name: Calcium peroxide, hydrogen peroxide, carbamide peroxide, and perhydrol urea

Dose: Brush as directed on package.

Brand names: Dazzzle, Dental White, EpiSmile, Instant White, Omni White & Bright, Rembrant Lighten, Ultimate White

Reasons: These agents work to whiten teeth in the same way that bleach acts on clothes to make them brighter.

Cautions: The safety of these agents has not been established and they must be tested further before they can be recommended for other than occasional use.

Brand Name Index

A

A-200 Pyrinate 144
A & D Ointment 134
Acephen Tablets, Suppositories 26, 28
Aceta 26
Acetaminophen Tablets, Drops, Suppositories, Uniserts 22, 24, 26, 28
Acid Mantel 137
Acne-Aid 114
Acnomel 114
Acnotex 114
Acromycin 121, 158
Actagen 72
Actidil Tablets, Liquid 71,161
Actifed 72
ACU-dyne Douche 123, 186
Acutrim 16 Hour Steady Control Tablets 196
Acutrim Late Day Tablets 196
Acutrim II Maximum Strength Tablets 196
Addaprin 162, 182

Adlerika 102
Adsorbotear 168
Advil 162, 182
Advil Cold & Sinus 60
aeroCaine 44, 125
aeroTherm 44, 125
Afko-Lube 109
Afrin 12-Hour Nasal 62
Afrin 12-Hour Pediatric 69
Aftate Cream, Gel, Powder, Spray 135, 141
After Burn Plus Gel, Spray 44, 125
Agoral 100
Akwa Tears 168
AK-Nefrin 171
Alamag 82
Alconefrin 25 & 50 62, 63
Aleve 20
Alka-Mints 82
Alka Seltzer 25
Alka-Seltzer Effervescent Antacid 85
Alka-Seltzer Extra Strength 26
Alka-Seltzer Flavored 25
Alkets 82

Kondremul with Phenolphthalein
   100
Konsyl 99
Konsyl-D 99

L

L.A. Formula 99
Lacril 168
Lagol 44, 125, 190
Lanabiotic Ointment 121, 135, 157
Lanacaine 44,125
Lanacane Aerosol, Cream 45, 94,
   190
Lanacort 45, 117, 146, 189
Lanoline 137
Laxcaps 100
Lax-Pills 101
Lice-Enz 144
Licetrol 144
Liqui-Doss 109
Liquifilm Forte 168
Liquifilm Tears 168
Liquiprin Children's 27
Liquiprin Elixir and Solution 22
Loperamide 91
Lotrimin AF Cream, Solution 140,
   160
Lubriderm 137

M

Maalox 83, 84
Maalox Anti-diarrheal 91
Maalox Anti-gas 89
Maalox Plus Extra Strength 83, 84
Maalox TC 83, 84
Magna Gel 83
Magnatril 84
Magnesia & Alumina 83
Mallamint 82
Marblen 82
Marezine 87
Marmine 88
Massengil MedicatedDisposable
   Douche 186
Massengil Med. Liquid 187
Massengil Vinegar & Water Dispos-
   able Douche 187

Measurin Timed Release 26
Meclizine 87
Meda Cap 27
Medicone Dressing 44, 125, 190
Medicone Rectal 93
Medihaler-Epi 77
Medipren 162, 182
Mediquell Chewy Squares 56
Medi-Quik 44, 121, 125, 135, 157
Merlenate 141
Metamucil (Instant & Flavored) 99
Mi-Acid 83
Micatin Cream, Powder, Spray 135,
   140, 160
Midol 26
Midol Maximum Strength 26
Midol PMS 185
Milk of Magnesia 102
Milroy Artificial Tears 168
Mintox 83
Mintox Plus 83
Mint Sensodyne 216
Mitrolan Chewable 99
Moisturel 137
Modane 101
Modane Bulk 99
Modane Mild 101
Modane Plus 100
Modane Soft 109
Moisture Drops 168
Monistat 7 191
Motrin IB 162, 182
Motrin IB Sinus 60
Multi-Symptom Menstrual Discom-
   fort Relief 185
Murine 168
Murine Ear Wax Removal System
   & Ear Drops 213
Murocel 167
Muro Tears 168
Myapap Drops 26
Mycelex-7 Cream, Tablets 191
Myciguent 121, 158
Myci-Spray 62
Mycitracin 121, 135, 157
Myfedrine Plus 72
Mygel 83
Mylanta 83, 84

Tarlene 149, 152
Tarsum 132
Tearguard 168
Tearisol 168
Tears Naturale 168
Tears Naturale II 168
Tears Plus 168
Tears Renewed 168
Tega Caine 44, 125
Tega Vert 88
Teldrin 71, 160
Tempra Chewable 26
Tempra Drops 26
Tempra Syrup 27
Tenol Plus 26, 27
Terramycin 121, 158
Tetrahydrozoline HCl 170
Therac 114
Therac-Plus 104
Therac-SB 104
TheraFlu Flu and Cold & Cough
    Medicine 67, 74
Theragran Jr. Children's Chewable
    Tablets 207
Theragran Jr. Children's Chewable
    Tablets with Extra Vitamin C
    207
Theragran Jr. with Iron Chewable
    Tablets 208
Theragran Tablets 207
Thinz-Back-To-Nature 197
Thinz Before Meals 198
Thinz-Span 197
Thorets 41
Tinactin 135, 141
Ting Cream, Powder, Spray 135, 141
Tirend Tablets 178
Tisit 144
Titracid 82
Titrilac 82
Trans-Ver-Sal 155
Triaminic Expectorant 59
Trigesic 26, 27
Trimycin 121, 135, 157
Triofed 72
Triphenyl Expectorant 59
Tri-pain 26, 27
Triple Antibiotic 121, 135, 157

Triple-X 144
Triptone 88
Tronolane Cream, Suppositories 94
Tums 82
Tums E-X 82
Tussex Cough 65
Ty-Cold 67
Tylenol Tablets, Drops, Elixir 24
Tylenol Allergy Sinus 74
Tylenol Childrens Tabs, Drops,
    Chewable, Elixir 22, 26, 27
Tylenol Cold No Drowsiness 66
Tylenol Extra Strength 27
Tylenol Multi-Symptom Cold 67
Tylenol PM 177
Tylenol Sinus Maximum Strength
    60

U V

Ultraprin 162, 182
Ultra Tears 168
Ultimate White 217
Unguentine Plus 44, 125
Unicap Capsules, Tablets 207
Unicap Jr. Chewable Tablets 207
Unicap Plus Iron Tablets 208
Unilax 100
Unitrol 198
Valadol 24
Valorin Super 27
Valprin 162, 182
Vanquish 26, 27
Vanseb 149, 152
Vanseb-T 132
Vaseline Dermatology Formula 137
Vaseline Pure Petroleum Jelly 134
VasoClear 171
Vick's Children's Cough 56
Vick's Throat Lozenges 41, 53
Vi-Daylin Chewable Tablets 206
Vi-Daylin Multi-vitamin Liquid 206
Vi-Daylin Plus Iron Liquid 207
Vigran Tablets 207
Viro-Med 67
Visine 171
Vivarin Tablets 178
V-Lax 99

Subject and Ingredient Index

Red Irritated Eyes 169
Rehydration 105
Respiratory Agents 52
Ringworm 140

S

Saccharin 199
Salicylic Acid 113, 126, 128, 130,
   148, 154
Scabies 150
Scrapes 157
Seborrhea 129, 151
Sedation 174
Selenium Sulfide 130
Senna 98
Simethicone 89
Sinus Congestion 56
Sinus Headache 59
Skin Protectants 133, 152
Skin Rash 70, 160
Sleep Aids 174
Sneezing 70
Sodium Bicarbonate 82
Sore Throat 35, 47, 52
Sprains 35
Stimulants 177
Stings 33, 47, 125
Stomach Ache 80
Stomach Acid 80
Stool Softeners 108
Strains 35
Strontium Chloride 215
Sulfur 113
Sunburn 35, 47, 153, 161
Suppositories 27, 103
Swelling (edema) 183
Swimmer's Ear 215

T

Talc 133
Tannic Acid 126
Teeth Desensitizers 215
Teething 35, 47
Teeth Whiteners 216
Tetracaine 93
Tetracycline 120, 157

Tetrahydrozoline 169
Theophylline 76
Throat 35, 47, 52
Tolnaftate 139
Toothache 36, 48
Topical Anesthetics 38, 116, 145
Topical Antiseptics 123
Topical Decongestants 61
Topical Steroid 45
Triprolidine 70

U

Ulcers 80
Undecylenic Acid 140

V

Vaginal Candidiasis 190
Vaginal Itch 45, 188
Vaginal Yeast Infection 197
Vegetable Oils 133
Vitamin Supplements 199
Vitamin C 209
Vitamin E 209
Viral Infection 31, 153
Vomiting 85, 86

W

Warts 153
Water Retention 183
Watery Eyes 70
Weight Control 193
Wheezing 77
Wounds 156

X

Xylometazoline 61

Y

Yeast Infections 158

Z

Zinc Oxide 93, 116, 133, 145
Zinc Pyrithione 130